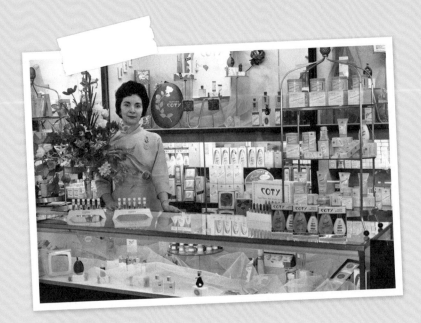

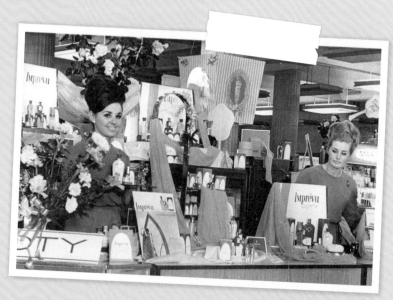

This book is dedicated to my
mum and nana.

INTRODUCTION

When I sat down to write the original copy for this book in 2019, I could never have imagined the response that it would receive. Number 1 on the *Sunday Times* Bestsellers list, the bestselling skincare book of all-time in the UK and winning Best Lifestyle Book at the British Book Awards in 2021. I don't think you can top that.

From the beginning my caveat to writing a skincare book was that I be allowed to keep it as up to date as possible. This industry changes so quickly, from legal advice on SPF, to new ingredients, to new formulas. It's vitally important to me that it remains relevant.

So, welcome to the
New Edit of *Skincare.*

I feel like I grew up in the industry. It's literally in my blood. Some of my earliest memories are of my grandmother religiously removing her makeup before bed. It was as hypnotising as it was methodical. Eyes first, in her bedroom mirror, then a full facial cleanse at the bathroom sink. The message was always the same: take care of your skin. It was non-negotiable. That message was passed down to my mum, who in turn made sure I heard it loud and clear. The first time I asked if I could buy some makeup, Mum said, 'Yes, once you've shown me you can take care of your skin.' That seemed a fair deal to get my hands on my first pot of Bourjois blush.

My nana started working on beauty counters in Liverpool in the 1960s, for Coty, then for Guerlain. We would go and meet her for lunch and the counter girls always looked immaculate, with their crisp uniforms, perfect makeup and styled hair. And they smelled amazing. My mum Cathy followed in her mother's footsteps, working for Coty as a teenager and going on to work for Helena Rubinstein in the 80s. As a teenager, I tried everything from white lipstick to blue eyeshadow, and Mum never batted an eyelid (though the black crimped hair and pale lipstick did make her look twice) — all she said was, 'Make sure you wash that off properly.'

It hadn't occurred to me to work in beauty until I'd had my first two children. I needed a part-time job and called my friend Lorraine, who at the time was working on the Aveda counter in Harvey Nichols. She'd always been the mate that I'd follow around London to buy my Clarins (I used Clarins pretty much throughout my late teens and early 20s). As it turned out, Aveda had a vacancy for a Saturday/Sunday salesperson. I went for the interview, got the job and never looked back. I realised on day two that not only was I good at the job, but that I loved it: I loved the interaction with customers, the banter on the shop floor, and the general retail environment. On reflection, I think I felt like I was also keeping up the family tradition. I discovered that I had a particular affinity with the skincare section. It made sense to me. One of my first staff training sessions sealed the deal: some of the tips and techniques that the trainer mentioned I still use to this day.

As much as I loved the shop floor, I knew I wanted to take my passion for skincare further. The Aveda counter had a beauty room attached to it and we were all trained in mini-treatments. I found I was trying to spend all of my time in the treatment rooms; it added another dimension to skincare that I found more interesting, to see it in action on someone's skin. I knew I wanted to qualify as a beauty therapist and that I had to go to the best training school available, with the highest qualification. I've always been annoyingly Type A.

> I started working for Space NK in London and knew 100 per cent that skincare was my thing.

And thanks to sitting through brand training sessions that would be either brilliantly informative or 'kill me now' dull, I learned how to talk to people if you want them to listen to you.

After doing my research and finding out what courses were available, I signed up to the prestigious Steiner Beauty School in Central London. They offered the best courses for me at the time, as they ran night classes, which meant I could keep working in the job I loved (and needed). I went to work as normal, then on Monday and Tuesday evenings I would go straight to class at Steiner, knocking up regular 50+-hour weeks while still being a wife and mother.

Steiner was brilliant. It was so old-fashioned, but the training – intense and in-depth – was excellent. They did not play: they were really strict and no-nonsense, and I loved it. I knew I had made the right choice. It took me longer to graduate than planned, as I had another two children while I was training. I would train as long as I could to clock up the required hours, go off and have a kid, then return to work full-time and head back to Steiner in the evenings, until I got the certificate that, without a doubt, sealed the direction that my career would eventually go in. It was hard, but when you're obsessed with what you're doing, and have an end goal, and support, it's fun. It also helps if your parents instilled a borderline-psychotic work ethic in you, which mine did. Thankfully.

I left Space NK and went on to work for Chantecaille and Liz Earle (among others), and at one point even did a stint at my beloved Clarins. The training was great – the uniform, not so much.

Eventually realising that I was a square peg in a round corporate hole, I started my own consulting business in 2009. My (at the time undiagnosed) ADHD would frequently land me in hot water as an employee, but as an independent consultant I was paid to tell brands what they needed to hear, not what they wanted to hear. As my husband once said, 'Who would have thought that being gobby and opinionated would become a career?'

When I started my blog in 2010, no one was really talking about skincare, and if they did, it was only to mention a new product release. The focus was very heavily on makeup and nails. My blog stood out. I could never have planned how successful it would become – you cannot 'make' something go viral.

I quickly gained a trusted audience by saying things like: 'Actually, I wouldn't advise that. Don't do that. Do this.' 'Don't put that on your face.' 'Wipes are horrible.' And so on. My followers are incredible, and insane about skincare.

The blog has now had over 200 million page views and has opened up a whole new world for me.

Through my Skincare Freaks Facebook group, I've seen every fad, heard every myth, and witnessed with my own eyes what works and what doesn't.

I've handled thousands of faces and tested so many products, and I'm lucky enough to count leading cosmetic scientists, the best dermatologists, expert doctors and especially my fellow aestheticians, as friends.

This book covers all issues for all ages, skin tones, budgets and skin types, from your daily routine to spots to dryness, and how to care for your skin when you're ill. You'll find tips to help you deal with pigmentation, dehydration, and lines and wrinkles, too.

I've taken everything I've learned from my years in the industry and my time on the blog to help you navigate the world of skincare simply and succinctly, tell you what you need and what you don't, and where not to waste your time and energy.

If I rave about a product or an ingredient, it's because I know it genuinely works.

Equally, if I say I'd like to push something off a cliff, it's because I know it's a waste of your hard-earned cash. If you already follow me, you'll be aware that I never kiss or blow smoke up anyone's arse – I haven't done it before and I'm not about to start now. And if you're new, welcome.

Thank you so much for reading. Skin Rocks™.

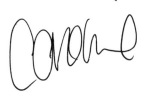

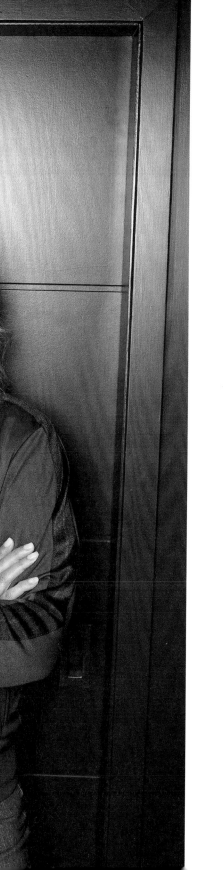

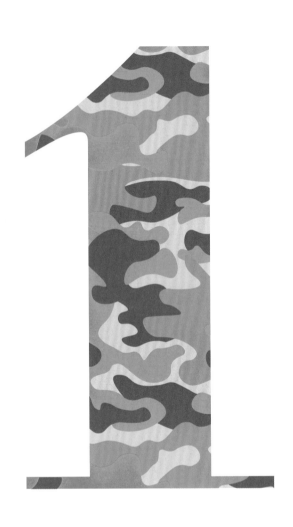

WHERE TO START !?#

"

SKIN
IS THE
FOUNDATION

"

WHERE TO START

Your skin is the biggest organ in your body, and it deserves a bit of attention. But that doesn't mean we all need to be scientists. Get into a few good habits with a daily routine and you'll soon see the benefits.

> A routine is the foundation of everything. And if you get it right, you can set your skin up for life.

Make it a habit. Morning and evening, for 2–3 minutes, or longer if you want to take the time to enjoy it. Make sure you take the time.

It's easy to see how your skincare routine can be a little overwhelming. We are sold so many products these days – there is something for everyone – but if you have more than two serums, which do you use first? And what about eye cream? And double cleansing and, and... stop. Chill. These pages explain exactly what needs to happen at each stage of your routine.

BEFORE WE BEGIN:

If it ain't broke, don't fix it. If you have a product that you've known and loved for a long time, and it works for you, I'm not telling you to change it. You know your skin best.

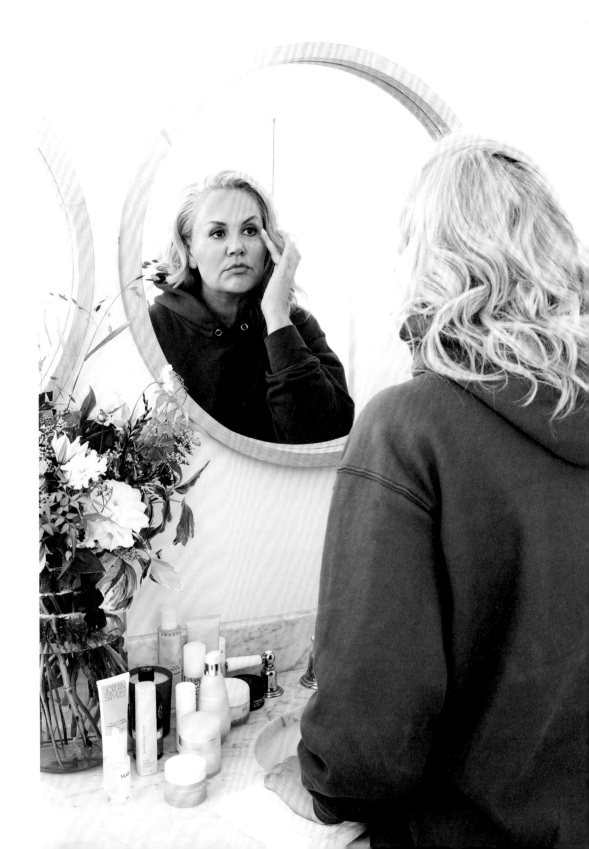

THE ESSENTIALS

Obviously everyone is different, but, *in general*, these are your basics if you're wondering where to start.

YOUR ROUTINE

- **Cleanse your skin every night without fail** – cleanliness is next to Godliness. Double cleanse if you are wearing makeup or sunscreen, or both (which applies to most of us).

  For those of you that say you have no time: either take your makeup off **as soon as you get home** OR **take your makeup off before you take your bra off** (if you sleep in your bra or don't wear one, then follow the first tip!).

- **Cleanse your skin every morning.** It obviously doesn't have to be as intense as the night-time cleanse, but a quick warm flannel and milk/balm/gel wouldn't go amiss to get rid of the overnight shedding. I know some brands say you don't need to cleanse your skin in the morning. That's okay. They're wrong.

- **TITTT: take it to the tits.** Your neck and décolleté, which is a fancy French term for your upper chest and shoulder area, are part of your facial skincare, too.

YOUR KIT

- **Use a high SPF daily** (30+, or 50+ on your face). Come rain or shine. Encourage your kids to use it, too. You will save them a lot of time trying to repair sun damage in later years.

- **Use good-quality skincare.** Choose your products wisely, not on the basis of discounts or trends.

- **Equate your skincare spending to what you would spend on a handbag or shoes.** I'm not saying you *should* – I'm saying you *should be willing to*.

- You're going to need to buy some **flannels or washcloths** (see page 25).

YOUR GROUND RULES

- **Wash your face properly.** A clean canvas makes everything better. There is no point in spending your hard-earned cash on expensive serums if you are using wipes or winging it when it comes to cleansing. See page 41 for more on cleansing.

- **Do not smoke.** That's really the beginning and end of it.

- **Get some sunshine.** The term 'everything in moderation' really applies here. I work indoors all day and live in the northern hemisphere. I don't get a lot of sun so I supplement with vitamin D (under doctor's advice). I don't use skincare with SPF: I apply it separately **in between** moisturiser and foundation or primer. SPF is too active an ingredient and can interfere with other anti-ageing ingredients, making all of your expensive moisturisers potentially redundant.

  Yes, obviously too much sun *is* damaging to the skin, but so is too much chlorine. And too much pollution. Get out there and get *some* sunshine. Some brands would have us believe the sun is the ultimate enemy. That's only true if you don't respect it. Get *some* sun. Not a lot, some. *Just don't be stupid about it.*

- **Get enough sleep.** When you are not getting sufficient rest, it shows on your face.

- **Try to eat well.** I'm not being a killjoy – a little of what you fancy definitely does you good – just don't go overboard. Gut health is linked to healthy skin function: for example, taking probiotics is thought to support a healthy skin.

- **Drink enough water.** This is important not only for the normal functionality of your skin, but for your general good health, too. If your urine is dark and you suffer from a lot of headaches, you would do well to up your H_2O levels.

- **Try to avoid stress.** I know it's much harder than it sounds, but do whatever you need to do to keep your stress levels low.

YOUR ROUTINE

I'm very aware that skincare can be intimidating. The aim of this book is to identify your skin's needs and choose your products accordingly.

The following pages will give you numerous options for products to use in your routine, broken into categories by age. This applies whatever your skin tone or gender.

If this is all new to you, it may appear confusing, unnecessary or even over the top. So, if you want to keep it basic and functional, you're looking for a good cleanser, moisturiser and SPF, **no matter your age**.

Consider the rest as guidance for how to manage a full routine if that's what you're looking for.

> Ultimately, your skincare kit can be as comprehensive or as simple as you want.

I was asked recently what I would take away with me if I could only pick three products. I went with a great balm cleanser, a good retinoid and an SPF50. If I had been asked the same question 30 years ago, I would have said a cleanser, a toner and a thick moisturiser. Your needs change with age, but if you are just starting out and are unsure of what you need, these are the basics.

TEENS – EARLY 20s

- A good eye-makeup remover. This can be from a chemist or a pharmacy brand and doesn't need to be expensive. If you don't wear much makeup, leave this out.

- A good cleanser. This can be your eye-makeup remover if funds are tight, but this age group traditionally embraces heavier makeup, so make sure you are removing it all properly.

- Consider an acid product if you suffer with acne or regular breakouts. Start with a mild lactic or salicylic acid. You do not need to use it every day. Glycolic is not necessary at this stage.

- A moisturiser or light hydrating lotion, depending on your skin type. This can be either a light lotion or a cream formula.

- SPF. Try to find an SPF50+ cream that feels comfortable on your skin. SPF30 is the absolute minimum you should go for. Regular use of an SPF at this age will save you time and money in later years.

ADD-ON:
A decent antioxidant – vitamin C serum is a safe bet. This isn't 100 per cent necessary as a teen, but it stands you in good stead for future years if you start in your early 20s.

20s – MID 30s

- A good eye-makeup remover or first cleanser.

- A second, lighter-textured cleanser for mornings or evenings where you aren't typically removing makeup or SPF.

- Acid toner. Using a gentle acid after your cleansing routine will help keep your skin exfoliated and ensure product penetration. You can introduce glycolic acid here, but lactic and salicylic acid are still helpful.

- A good antioxidant serum. Vitamin C and niacinamide are both good options.

- A multi-molecular-weight hyaluronic acid serum. As you are nearing or entering your 30s, your skin will slowly start to find it more challenging to retain oil and water. Hyaluronic acid is your best friend.

- Eye product. Optional if budget restricts, more necessary if you wear glasses or if your face is regularly exposed to the sun.

- A vitamin A/retinol product. This is not a concern if you are fairly healthy and don't sunbathe/smoke etc., however, if you are the other side of 30 and do, you need a retinoid.

- A moisturiser suited to your skin type.

- SPF. Same as earlier years. Use SPF50+, or at least a minimum of SPF30.

ADD-ONS:
A light facial oil if you feel you need it, or in the winter. Apply a couple of drops under your moisturiser in the morning or finish with it in your evening routine. A hydrating hyaluronic-based facial mist. This will keep your hydration levels topped up in the skin without the added weight of a heavier cream.

LATE 30s – EARLY 40s

- A good eye-makeup remover or first cleanser.

- A lighter-textured cleanser for your morning cleanse or evenings as a second cleanse, where you aren't typically removing makeup or SPF.

- Acids. Glycolic, lactic or PHA acids can all make an appearance in your kit at this stage, depending on your skin's needs (see pages 122–129).

- A hyaluronic-based facial mist. Your skin finds it harder to retain moisture at this age – this spray replaces that lost moisture. Do not spray plain water over your face: it is not the same thing. Look for 'hyaluronic acid' on the product.

- A good antioxidant serum. Spend your money here. Get a good niacinamide/vitamin C/resveratrol etc., and use it daily.

- A good-quality hyaluronic product. You are more susceptible to trans-epidermal water loss (TEWL) at this age so you will benefit from a daily dose of hyaluronic acid. Do not be fooled into buying a dirt-cheap one: it's likely to be a single-ingredient, heavy hyaluronic acid that won't really penetrate, so it's a false economy.

- Facial oil. Your quickest fix and your best friend.

- Eye product. You will notice the need for these more at this age. Go for lighter textures like gels or light creams. Rich, thicker creams feel luxurious but will make your eyes puffy.

- Vitamin A/retinoid. A must.

- A moisturiser suited to your skin type.

- SPF. Do not forgo this critical step.

40s, 50s, 60s, 70s, 80s & 90s

- A good eye-makeup remover or first cleanser. You may prefer thicker cream cleansers at this point.

- A second, lighter-textured cleanser for mornings or evenings where you aren't typically removing makeup or SPF.

- Acids. Glycolic, lactic and PHA acids are all great for older skins.

- A hyaluronic-based facial mist, to replace lost moisture.

- Eye products. Go for gels if you have crepey eyes, or light creams. Richer eye creams are not favourable on an older face.

- Vitamin A/retinoid. An absolute must. Your skin's cell turnover is extremely slow at this age. Vitamin A is your best friend. Jump in.

- Facial oil. A facial oil will prove beneficial if you know that menopause has made your skin much drier than it used to be. It will literally replace the glow on an older face.

- Good antioxidant serums. While these are still important, you may prefer to spend your money 'correcting' issues at this age, and that brings us to...

- A good-quality pigmentation serum/product.

- A good-quality hyaluronic product.

- A moisturiser suited to your skin type. You may want to spend a little more on a moisturiser at this age. There is some merit to a separate night cream for an older skin, but it's more of a 'nice to have' product than a must.

MORNING ROUTINE

The main point of the morning routine is to prep your skin for the day.

Taking care of your skin in the morning is no different to having a shower before you put clean knickers on.

You may think this is obvious, but I am contacted regularly by people who say, 'Do I really need to cleanse in the mornings?' Yes.

I don't know about you, but I wake up with a lovely glow in the mornings – maybe you do too?

It's called sweat. Please wash your face.

SHOWER FIRST

I have never put my face under the shower. The water is too hot for your face (well, my choice of water temperature certainly is). You also have the surfactants from your shampoo running all over your face. Stand with your back to the shower and your chin raised – like the shower has greatly offended you.

Cleanse when you get out of the shower, not before.

FLANNELS

Flannels get your skin CLEAN. Think of your parents: how did they wash you when you were a kid? They used a flannel.

They are more substantial than wipes or muslin, are far more effective at removing dirt, and help exfoliate the skin, too.

Buy eight flannels minimum and use one a day (you'll need the eighth flannel as a spare on wash day): start with a fresh, clean flannel for your morning cleanse and use the same flannel for your evening cleanse, chucking it in the washing basket when you're done.

You don't have to spend a fortune on the plushest, fluffiest flannels. Any will do. But go for white so you get the satisfaction of seeing the muck come off.

Machine-wash your flannels so they get properly clean, but avoid using fabric softener, as traces can end up on your skin.

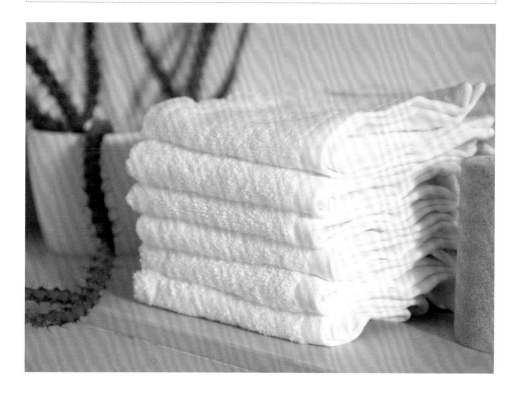

MORNING ROUTINE

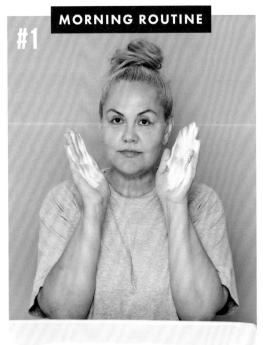

#1

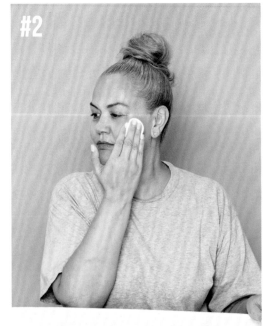

#2

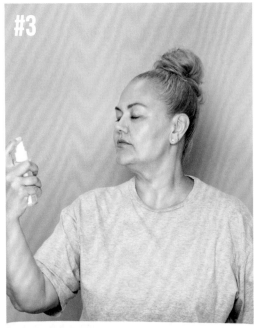

#3

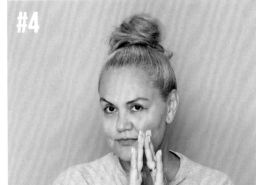

#4

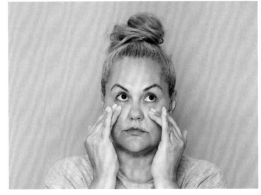

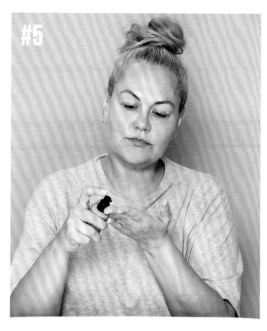

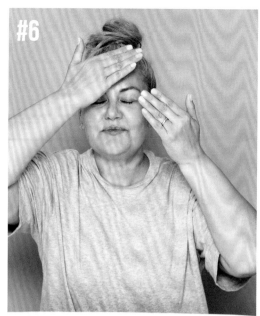

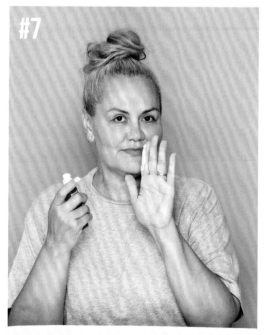

STEP-BY-STEP

1 Use your hands to apply your cleanser. Wipe off the cleanser with a clean, warm, damp flannel.

2 Exfoliate your skin with an acid toner or acid wipe.

3 Spray your skin with a hydrating spray.

4 Put a little cream on the edge of your ring finger, blend it with the other ring finger, then apply to the eyes. You need enough to cover the entire orbital area, over and below your eye.

5 Put a couple of drops of serum or facial oil on your fingertips, then use the fingertips of the other hand to apply immediately.

6 Apply moisturiser all over your face, neck and décolletage: take it to the tits. Your skin should feel comfortable, not 'wet'.

7 Apply at least one finger-length SPF after your moisturiser, and make sure you use enough.

#CLEANSE

Milk, balm (a little), gel, foaming (the newer types) – as long as it doesn't turn your face into a foam bath, carry on. Yes, you can absolutely use the same product in the morning that you use in the evening if you want to, but you're only cleansing once.

Use a clean flannel.

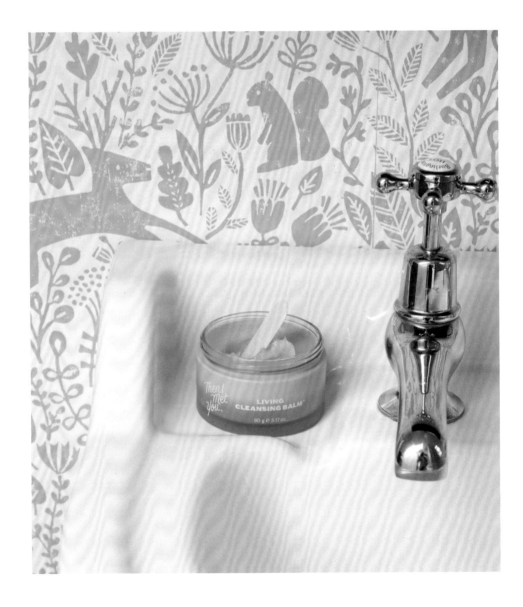

#EXFOLIATE

Rather than harsh scrubs (which are thankfully going out of fashion), acids are about taking off the layer of dead skin cells and, depending on the type of acid, stimulating the skin. **Your skin's surface is naturally acidic, and acid toners lower your skin's pH.** They have the effect of blowing a trumpet in your ear. Your skin is forced into action.

Most brands make exfoliating/acid products that you use at the traditional 'toner' stage. To call them a 'toner' is to do them a great injustice – these are the 'toners' of the 21st century.

Try to have a couple of exfoliating/acid products if you can: a milder version and a more 'active' one. There's no point in having two of one type. Alternate them daily. There are lots of different types of acids (see pages 122–129) but the main ones are glycolic, lactic and salicylic. If you can only afford one, either buy a mild one and use it twice a day, or a stronger one and use it in the evenings only. If you have sensitive skin, or you are just concerned about using acids, start by using them twice a week and see how your skin reacts.

All packaging for *anything* with *any* acid in it will legally have to say 'avoid eye area'. Unless you are using a prescription strength, dermatologist-prescribed hardcore acid, it's fine. Apply the acidic toner on cotton pad or gauze then take it around the eyes – full circle – upper brow to corner brow and under eye to inner eye – and reverse.

Caveat: using acids twice a day or even daily may be too much or unnecessary for some skins, especially if you are also using active ingredients (see page 248) in other products, such as strong retinoids in the evenings. If you're new to acids, start slowly and follow your skin's response.

Go easy and listen to your skin. If you have overdone it or your skin feels like you've gone too far, acid is the first thing you should drop. Actives are the second.

#SPRAY HYDRATE

I love this step. It's the start of the hydrating process and it wakes me up. Use whatever hydrating flower mist or water you like. Any spray should have glycerin or hyaluronic acid in there somewhere, but something like a good-quality rosewater is fine. I mean *good* quality – i.e. the INCI (International Nomenclature of Cosmetic Ingredients – see Glossary pages 284–293) list is proper rosewater, not fragrance (parfum) and colouring. Check your ingredient labels.

You can also use your traditional 'toner' at this stage, as long as its main function is to hydrate. Some traditional toners are designed to 'mattify' or strip back sebum (see Glossary) and this is not what we want. If you are using toner in this way, decant it into a spray bottle and keep it as a spray, too. Try to avoid alcohol at this stage.

#APPLY EYE PRODUCT

Do not apply your eye product last. No matter how carefully you apply your serums and moisturisers you will always get some in the eye area, and then your eye product won't be absorbed where you want it to be. Pointless.

Apply eye products to the orbital area (the area covered by your sunglasses) before serum, moisturiser and SPF (you can put these on top of the eye product if you fancy it and it's not a contraindication).

"

APPLYING YOUR EYE PRODUCT LAST IS LIKE WEARING YOUR KNICKERS OVER YOUR TROUSERS

"

#APPLY SERUM

This step is what I am asked about the most. Application goes by texture. Water-based serums should be applied first, followed by oil-based serums. It is worth highlighting however, that heavier oil-based serums can disrupt your SPF, so I tend to use those in the evenings wherever possible. Spending 20 seconds 'warming' your serum in your hands by rubbing them together is a complete waste of time, money and product, unless your intention is to have fabulously soft palms (see pages 48–49 for my 'therapist hands' technique for dispersing product in the palms and onto the fingers).

There will *always* be exceptions, so if what you are doing works for you, don't change it on my account.

#MOISTURISE

Choose your moisturiser according to your skin *type*, not skin *condition*. Your moisturiser is your coat/protection. People tend to spend far too long choosing their moisturiser and far too little time taking care of what goes on beforehand: for example, using a quick swipe of a wipe, slapping on an expensive face cream and then wondering why their skin isn't great.

Remember to avoid anything 'mattifying' – a promise that's often made on products for oily skin. Skin is not designed to be 'matte'.

Your skin has plenty of time to be matte when you're dead.

If your skin is excessively oily, just go for light hyaluronic acid serums, which help lock in moisture, and oil-free moisturisers. No need to force the issue. Leave that to your makeup.

Whatever moisturiser you are using that is right for your skin, whack it on now.

!?#

YOUR SKIN 'SLEEPS' DURING THE DAY

No. Your skin does not, will not, and has never 'slept' during the day.

The other argument for using different products in the evening is that your skin 'may' relax a little while it's not busy fighting off free radicals (see Glossary). Funnily enough, free radicals are not particularly conscious of time and are, in fact, around us 24/7, but that's apparently by-the-by for some marketing people. If you wanted to really annoy someone you could argue that as soon as you breathe out carbon dioxide, your face is surrounded by a cloud of free radicals.

You use different products at night because you don't need SPF (or thicker 'protecting' moisturisers), which means you can use lighter, more effective formulations – serums/oils/retinoids etc. – to target and treat skin issues.

AM: Protect
PM: Treat and repair

'Your skin is your biggest organ.' Replace the word 'skin' in this sentence with 'heart', 'brain', 'lungs', 'kidney' or 'liver' and see how long you would be alive for.

'Your skin sleeps during the day'?
Right, well, that's me dead then.

#APPLY SPF

Apply one finger-length of SPF to your face, and apply more if you know you haven't sufficiently covered an area (see page 154 for more on product quantities).

Make sure you also apply your SPF everywhere, including the back of your neck and the top of your ears. Women typically apply their SPF before they hit the beach and put their hair in a ponytail the minute they hit the sand. EARS! Even if you aren't on holiday.

For more on SPF and why it is essential, see page 146.

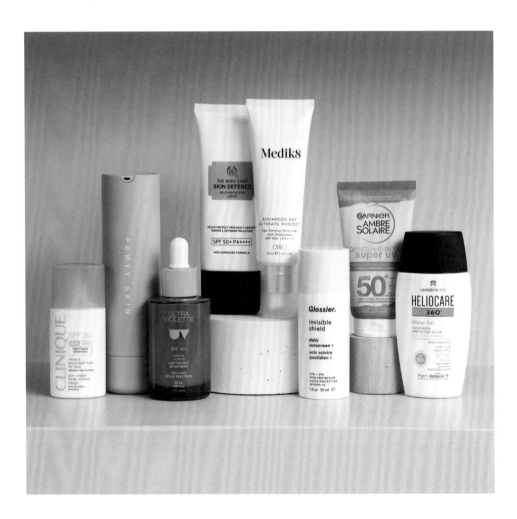

!?#

IF YOU HAVE OILY SKIN YOU DO NOT NEED TO MOISTURISE

The biggest mistake people with oily/combination skin make is to try to 'strip' the skin during the cleansing stage – to the point where it squeaks *faints* – and then not apply anything else on top and just go.

Your face is not a shampoo advert. You cannot just 'wash'n'go'.

For the more lubricated among us:

#1   Cleanse your face with a good cleanser. This could be oil, cream, milk, gel or foaming – just no 'washing up liquid' foaming ingredients (SLS) please.

#2   Exfoliate with an acidic toner.

#3   Spray hydrate.

#4   Apply a light serum to target specific skin conditions (ageing, pigmentation, scarring/dehydration etc.) if that is a concern.

#5   Apply either a hyaluronic serum, a moisturiser, or in the evening, even a facial oil designed for your skin type.

> Use serums to treat your skin **condition**. Use moisturisers or facial oils to treat your skin **type**.

Washing your face and going out with nothing on it is akin to leaving the house butt naked.

ROUTINE AFTER EXERCISING

I am frequently asked by people that exercise in all manner of ways about when they should schedule their skincare routines and what they should use. As there are SO many variations, I thought I'd try to cover all bases.

So, let's start with the 'skeleton' or bare bones.

JOGGING/RUNNING

Early-morning run:

COLD CLIMATE (ENGLISH WINTER FOR EXAMPLE)
Apply a little facial oil to protect your face before you pound the streets, go run, sweat, come home, do morning skincare routine.

HOT CLIMATE
Apply SPF before you hit the streets, go run, come home, do skincare routine.

After-work run:

Remove makeup, apply a thin layer of moisturiser (and/or SPF if outside and the sun is out), go run, sweat, shower, do your proper evening skincare routine.

GYM SESSIONS/WEIGHTS/CARDIO

Early-morning classes:

Get up, if you have dry skin apply a little moisturiser, go to the gym, sweat it out in your class/workout, shower, then do your proper morning skincare routine.

Lunchtime classes:

Go to the gym, remove your makeup, apply a minimal moisturiser (a thin layer), do your class/workout, sweat like a racehorse, shower, repeat your morning skincare routine.

After-work classes:

Go to the gym, remove makeup and apply a thin layer of light moisturiser, do your class/workout, sweat, shower, then do your full evening skincare routine – unless you're going out for dinner etc., in which case apply moisturiser, apply your makeup and remove it all before bed as usual.

SWIMMING

It's not great to swim in makeup, no matter how rushed you are. Equally, you don't want a ton of moisturiser (or other product) running into your eyes and blinding you while you do your laps.

Early-morning swim:

Get up, apply a thin layer of moisturiser (I avoid my forehead to prevent product dripping down into the eyes, but do what you feel your skin needs), swim, shower, do morning skincare routine.

After-work swim:

Remove makeup, put on a thin layer of something protective – I prefer a little facial oil, but light moisturiser works – swim, shower, do your full evening skincare routine, unless you're going out for dinner.

CYCLING

Whatever time of day you cycle, you want protection on a face that is being wind-bashed. Cycle with no makeup, make sure you have applied a protective moisturiser and/or SPF, and do your full skincare routine after your post-cycle shower. I would consider applying facial oil to the cheeks too, although you might end up covered in bug roadkill.

HOT YOGA

Being frank, hot yoga is not good for your face. The entire purpose of it is to make you sweat, however, unlike in other sports, you can't cool down because you're in a room where the temperature is maintained at 'scorching'. That healthy 'glow' will eventually lead to broken capillaries. Having said that, I know some of you are completely addicted to it, so your main concern is to keep the nose/cheek area under control.

> It should go without saying that you should not be wearing a full face of makeup for exercise, ever.

After the class, spritz as soon as you can with a floral water – not normal water – shower, then apply a hydrating serum AND moisturiser. You will be dehydrated afterwards, so if you regularly attend hot yoga classes I would keep spritzing bottles handy, and keep an eye on your face for signs of dehydration like fine lines and cakey makeup.

EXERCISE + SKINCARE TIPS

- Remove your makeup before you exercise. Yes, you can use micellar water if you have to, but you would be much better off using a good oil cleanser: it's more gentle and nourishing and kinder all round, especially if you exercise every day, or four to five times a week.

Try to exercise with a light moisturiser on your face.

- If you are going to use saunas and steam rooms, have some facial oils on your face – heat and oils are lovely. Don't use a mineral oil-based product on this occasion – go for plant oils instead. (A paraffin wax mask done by a professional is great, but that's because it is done by a pro with a good plant oil underneath.)

- Protect the cheeks: those are the areas most prone to visible signs of damage from sport. Use oils, moisturisers and SPF where appropriate.

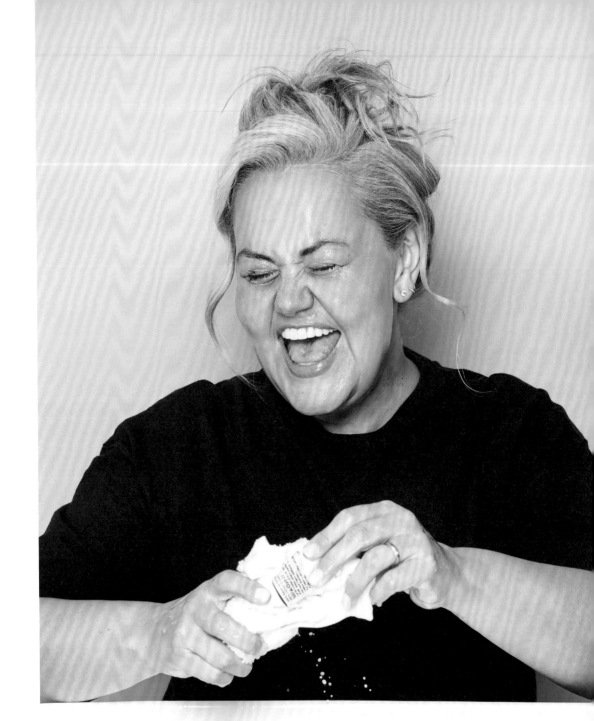

EVENING ROUTINE

> At home? Bra off. Hair up.
> Clean your face.

The main point of your evening routine is to help your skin help itself.

Repair and correct.

Your face is not being bombarded with sunlight, dirt, aggressors etc. at night, so you can get the treatments in while they actually have a better chance of being effective.

'Your skin repairs itself at night' is the biggest old wives' tale out there in skincare. It's nonsense. And please don't get me started on **'Your skin sleeps at night'**. No. YOU sleep at night. Your skin does not have an on/off switch like your heating. **Your skin is repairing itself 24 hours a day** – the reason you use treatments while you sleep is *because you have the full attention of your skin.*

#CLEANSE

'Do I need to double cleanse?' is my most frequently asked question about the evening routine. The only time I don't double cleanse is if I have been indoors all day and have applied neither SPF nor makeup. Otherwise, I go straight in with an oil-based product to hit the grease, dirt, makeup and general gunk on my face after a day in Central London.

If you wear SPF you need to double cleanse. A lot of people who think they are allergic to SPF because it breaks them out are simply not taking the time to wash it off properly. (Please don't take it personally if you genuinely are allergic to SPF – I'm clearly not talking to you.)

SPF is designed to stay on your face.
Take the time to remove it.
Makeup is designed to stay on your face.
Take the time to remove it.

Using the flannel from the morning is fine. I usually use two out of the three products below.

- Pre-cleanse oil or eye-makeup remover
- Oil/balm cleanser
- Milk/gel cleanser

NOTE TO MICELLAR WATER USERS: if you prefer to take your makeup off with a micellar water before you cleanse, that is your first cleanse. But if you are wearing an SPF or heavy makeup you still need to go a couple of rounds with a flannel. Don't be lazy. Your skin will thank you.

#APPLY VITAMIN A

If you are using vitamin A (see pages 136–137), apply it onto dry skin after cleansing. Leave it for about 20 minutes, then follow it with your eye product. If you need it, apply your moisturiser afterwards. If you are new to vitamin A, or are using a strong vitamin A product, the effects can be quite extreme at first so you may need to buffer it by applying a moisturiser or mild facial oil around 20–30 minutes after applying it.

IT'S OKAY TO SLEEP IN YOUR MAKEUP

Enough already.

STOP SAYING that it is okay to sleep in your makeup. It is not. The average woman wears a mix of the following:

- SPF
- Primer
- Foundation
- Powder
- Concealer
- Blusher
- Bronzer
- Eyeshadow (multiple)
- Eyeliner
- Mascara
- Brow pencil
- Lip liner
- Lipstick
- Lip gloss

That is a LOT of product on your face. SPF, in particular, is designed to stick to your face; that's its job. Add to that all the dirt and pollution from being outside and you have the perfect storm brewing for spots, dehydration, dullness – a whole plethora of issues.

Wash your face at night.
Do not sleep in your makeup.

If your partner prefers you with makeup, get a new partner. 😉

#APPLY EYE PRODUCT

As in the morning routine, if you typically wake up with puffy eyes, move to a lighter texture and use a serum or gel. Avoid rich creams.

#APPLY TREATMENT PRODUCTS (USUALLY SERUMS) OR FACIAL OILS

This is my favourite step. This is where you can really go to town. **Treatment products should be your main expense skincare-wise.** Try to have at least three products you can use, depending on your skin's needs. *At least.*

Use a good facial oil, a good serum or treatment – whatever you need for your skin. And before you ask me what you need, really think about it. You know your skin.

Whether or not you use a night-time moisturiser depends on what treatment you use. If your treatment is IN your moisturiser, you're done. If you are using a lovely night-time oil, you may not want/need anything else. Personally, I am a fan of the 'piling it on lightly' approach.

> All this 'cleanse and then just let your skin breathe' is daft. Your skin is always breathing. If it wasn't, you'd soon know about it. In the morgue.

Your skin will breathe regardless of whether you put product on it or not.

My PM routine is literally: pre-cleanse, cleanse, acid, spray hydrate, eye product, oil/treatment and night treatment/oil/cream (not all three!).

Sometimes less is really not more. Having one cleanser and one moisturiser is like having one pair of shoes or one bra. If you can afford more than one pair of shoes, you can afford more than one cleanser and more than one moisturiser.

'WARM PRODUCT IN HANDS BEFORE USE'

This is another thing that brands have got into the habit of putting on their packaging.

A good formulation will be ready to go as soon as it comes out of the bottle or tube, so warming a product in your hands will only put most of the product on your hands. Oil doesn't need to be warmed to be absorbed. If you want to rub it in your hands and inhale it before you apply it, that's your choice, but it won't change the way it works.

> I prefer to put the product on my face and smell it while it gets to work on my face – not my hands.

If your product is such that it needs to be 'warmed', I probably wouldn't bother. As always, there are some exceptions: Weleda Dry Skin Food, for example, needs a little help.

My 'therapist hands' technique (see pages 48–49) shows you how to apply your product so you see the benefits on your face, rather than your hands.

#1

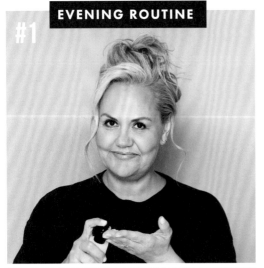

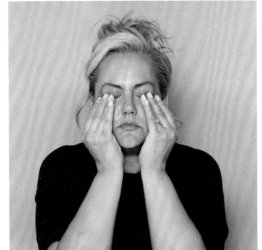

#2

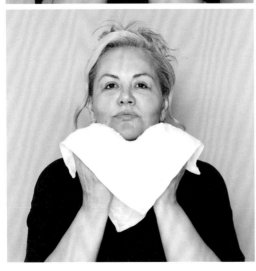

#3

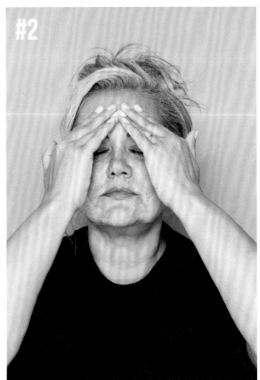

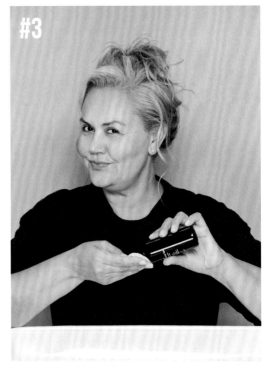

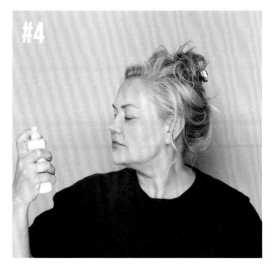

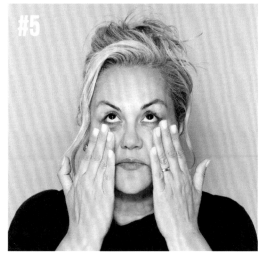

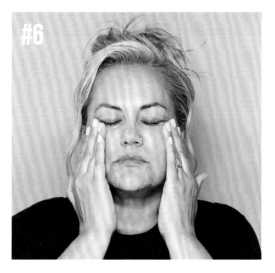

1 If you have been wearing SPF and/or makeup, you need to double cleanse.

If you're wearing lots of eye makeup, swipe around the eyes with a cleansing oil, using your fingertips, or use a dedicated eye-makeup remover on cotton pads if you're wearing lash extensions or a lot of mascara.

Get your cleansing oil or balm straight on and around the eye area first, then spread it out across the rest of the face. To take it off, hold a flannel under a warm running tap, squeeze out excess water, then wipe away makeup. (Don't fill the sink bowl with water – this cleansing stage will not splash off.)

2 If you have only done one cleansing step at this stage, finish with a quick going over of a lighter milk or gel cleanser geared for your skin type. Get it straight onto the skin, then off with a warm, damp flannel.

3 Apply either acid toner or vitamin A (optional). If using vitamin A, you would normally apply onto dry skin after cleansing (although some brands, and I, would recommend applying to damp skin for deeper penetration). Leave it for about 20 minutes, then follow with eye product.

If you're not using a vitamin A product, proceed as in the morning routine (without SPF).

4 Spray your skin with a hydrating spray

5 Apply eye product as in the morning routine.

6 Apply your treatments, facial oils or moisturisers (but you don't need all three).

47

Don't forget to put your flannel in the wash!

APPLYING PRODUCT

One of the things I see time and again is people spending ages warming and rubbing skin products into their hands rather than putting them to work on their face! Why?! This technique makes sure the product gets onto your face. I call it 'therapist hands' because no professional would put expensive product on their hands and spend time rubbing it into their palms before applying it. You should not need to warm a product in your hands to make it work (see page 45).

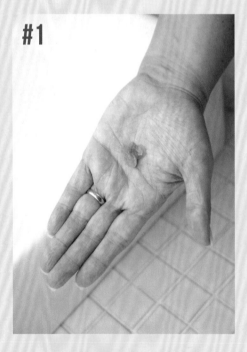

#1

Deposit product into the centre of your palm.

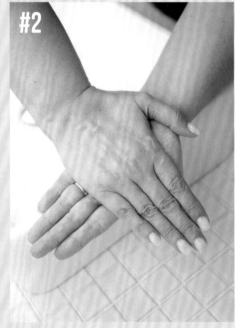

#2

Put your palms together in an 'X'.

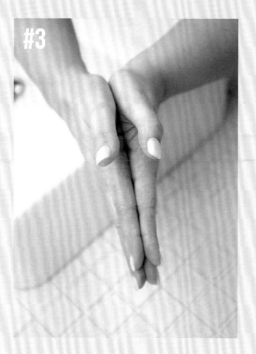

#3

Twist the hands 90 degrees so that your palms are facing.

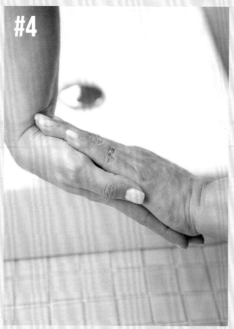

#4

Twist the hands a further 180 degrees so that your palms are opposing.

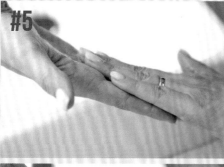
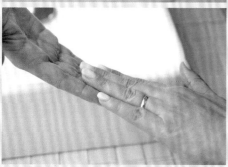

#5

Pull your hands apart smoothly.

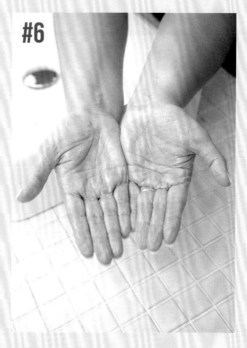

#6

The product should be evenly distributed across your fingers and palms ready for application.

HOW MUCH PRODUCT SHOULD I USE?

Take this as a rough guide, not hard-and-fast rules: everyone's face is different in size (mine is huge!). Remember the mantra: *grip, not slip.* Your face shouldn't feel greasy or slippery.

CLEANSER

First cleanse/makeup removal – balm: either a big fat grape or two grapes if they're smallish [1].

First cleanse/makeup removal – milk: a heaped teaspoon or two pumps (if applicable) [2].

Second cleanse/AM cleanse – a level teaspoon (or one pump, if applicable).

ACID TONING

Dampen a flat cotton pad (not cotton-wool balls) until two thirds of the pad is wet. Use both sides. Always. For pre-soaked pads, use one pad on both sides.

EYE PRODUCT

I usually use about a 'pine nut' per eye. If your eyes are dry or showing signs of ageing, then you may want slightly more. But for younger skins, one pine nut on the edge of your ring finger, blended with the opposing finger then applied to the eyes, is sufficient. You need enough to cover the entire orbital area, over and below your eye.

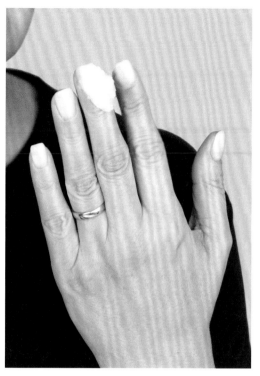

CLEANSER 1

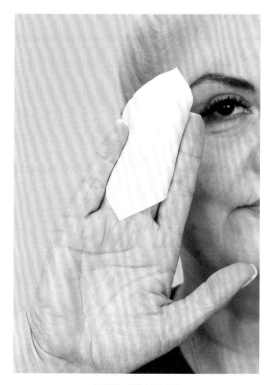

CLEANSER 2

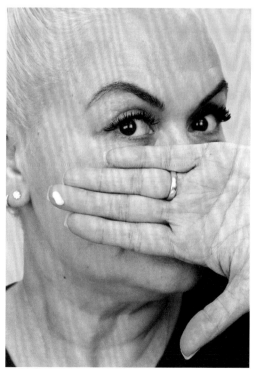

ACID TONING

EYE PRODUCT

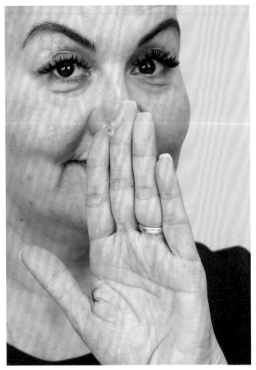

SERUMS

MOISTURISER / NIGHT CREAM

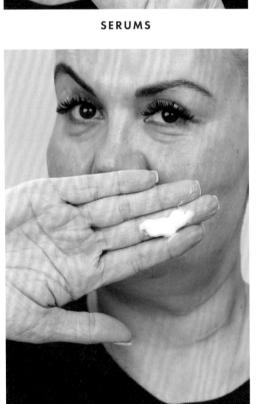

SPF

SERUMS

Serums are easy to gauge because the majority of them are in a bottle fitted with a dispensing pump and are designed to be dispensed at one pump per application. Ergo, if you have a large face, use two pumps, and for a smaller face, use one pump. For comparison purposes, about the size of an almond.

There has, however, been a huge increase in the use of pipettes for serums (I hate them – they are messy to use, you're more likely to drop them and waste product, and they allow air into the formula). If yours has a pipette, start with half a pipette maximum, adding a little more if you need it.

MOISTURISER AND NIGHT CREAM

Depending on your skin and face size, two blueberries, or three if you're a dry pumpkin head. Think almond-size again.

SPF

To achieve the SPF on the label, you need 2 milligrams of sunscreen per square centimetre.

The official recommendations change regularly, but the current thinking is for the face, you apply two full finger-lengths of SPF.

I think that can be too much for some, after all, we all come in different sizes, so start with one full finger-length, and apply more if you know you haven't sufficiently covered an area.

WHAT TO USE DAILY AND WHAT TO DIP IN AND OUT OF

Now that you have established the foundations of a good routine, you should have a better idea of which products you need to use when. And, of course, what to look out for if you have particular needs. Whether you're tweaking a routine you already had, or finally throwing out the face wipes and giving your skin the TLC it deserves, you may have identified some gaps in your routine and be looking for some new products.

The volume of products out there is huge, and when there's always something new and exciting on the market, sometimes you want to give it a try. But some products are designed to be used continually until you reach the end of the bottle, and won't benefit from being put back on the shelf too soon. So, what should you 'use up' quickly and when is it okay to mix and match?

In general, use up your middle (serums, oils) and dabble with your bookends (cleanser, moisturiser).

- **Cleansers.** You can mix up cleansers. Go by what you're wearing on your skin – makeup or SPF, whether it's a morning or evening cleanse, and your skin type or current skin condition (see Skin Types and Conditions chapter). Equally, it's totally and completely fine to own and use just one.

- **Eye products.** Choose one and use it up before buying another. Having said that, eyes are usually the first place to tell you if they aren't happy with a product. Eye products are not something you 'persevere' with. If it doesn't suit your skin, pass it on.

- **Acids.** These generally keep for a healthy period of time due to their preservative qualities, so using a couple of different ones a week shouldn't do any harm, although try to remember to use different types of acids as opposed to just different types of the same acids: most people, when asked, turn out to have two or three glycolic acids, but no lactic or salicylic. Lactic acid is a safe starting point for most people if you haven't used an acid before (see page 122).

- **Serums.** These should absolutely be used until finished up, especially vitamin Cs, retinoids etc. When they're empty, you can work out if your skin liked the product/you saw a noticeable improvement and if you need to step it up or move back a gear.

- **Moisturiser.** While it's nice to have lots of moisturisers, they're unnecessary. These days I tend to finish the moisturiser I'm using before moving on to a new one. I do have ones for drier days, and ones for travelling, but generally I get through them in a pretty methodical fashion.

- **SPF.** The best SPF is one that you are going to use. Find one you like and use it daily. Don't 'keep' SPFs from one holiday to the next. They degrade.

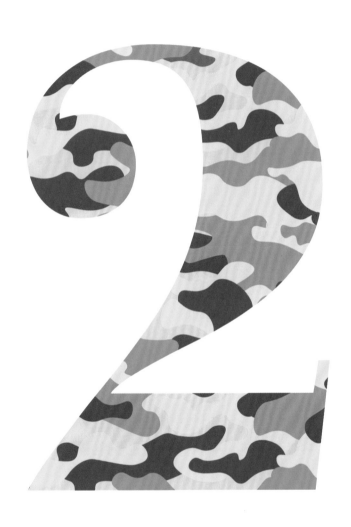

KNOW YOUR SKIN

HOW SKIN WORKS

Your skin is incredible. Whether you're a bright young thing without a wrinkle in sight, someone who's struggled with acne their entire lives, or an older person in the first flushes of menopause wondering what the hell's going on with your complexion, your skin is still a miracle of nature. It's hard at work every day underneath all the grease, sweat, dirt, pollution, makeup and gunk.

In fact, **your skin is the biggest organ in your body.** It's a living, breathing mechanism and it's working overtime for you. These are just a few of the jobs it's doing, 24 hours a day:

- Acting as a waterproof shield so that vital nutrients don't leak out of your body (gross).

- Regulating your temperature, by opening and closing blood vessels, and perspiring to allow sweat to evaporate and cool us down.

- Acting as a barrier between your insides and the many harmful toxins and microorganisms in the environment.

- Sweating out waste products, including salt and ammonia.

- Helping protect you from sun damage by producing melanin.

- Synthesising vitamin D for strong bones and healthy organs.

- Patching itself up against the various cuts, bruises, grazes and burns that we get day to day.

- Giving us that little thing known as the sense of touch, which we'd be pretty screwed without.

It's complex, and it deserves respect. To understand how your skincare products work, it can help to have a basic understanding of what goes on beneath your skin.

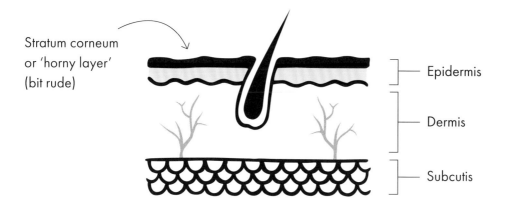

Stratum corneum or 'horny layer' (bit rude)

Epidermis

Dermis

Subcutis

EPIDERMIS

This is the outermost part of the skin, and the bit that you see. It's made up of keratinocytes (our skin cells), and is the part of you that keeps bacteria at bay. It's your first line of defence.

Your epidermis is constantly renewing and regenerating, with new cells made in the lowest layer, the basal cells, and travelling, over the course of about a month, to the top. The 'living' layers of cells are known as the 'squamous cells', which eventually become a layer of dead keratinocytes that are constantly shedding in the stratum corneum. This process slows down as you get older. So, making sure you're keeping your skin clean and exfoliated is important if you don't want your complexion to look dull and lifeless.

The bottom layer of the epidermis also produces melanin, which helps protect you from UV rays and gives your skin its colour. When you tan, your skin is actually producing more melanin in an attempt to shield you from the sun.

Over-the-counter skincare will only ever treat the epidermis. If you want to go deeper, you'll need a prescription or a needle.

THE DERMIS

This thicker layer of your skin contains the blood vessels and nerves that give you your sense of touch. The connective tissues are made up of two proteins: collagen, which gives skin its fullness and shape; and elastin, which gives skin its resilience and its ability to 'snap' back into shape. The cells that make these proteins are bathed in hyaluronic acid, a cellular lipid that holds water and gives your skin its bounce and texture.

When you are young, the dermis is so full of collagen and elastin that it can bounce back into shape, but as we age, they break down faster than our cells can replace them, and this leads to wrinkles and dry skin.

The dermis also contains your hair follicles and oil glands, as well as the beginning of your pores, which push hair, sweat and oil to the surface.

SUBCUTANEOUS TISSUE

This is a layer of fat and tissue lying between your skin and muscles. It protects your muscles from the beating your skin gets every day, and insulates and regulates your body's temperature too.

The subcutaneous tissue layer tends to thin as we age, and when this happens our skin looks less smooth, and the underlying veins show through. It also results in cellulite in other areas of the body.

Nobody's asking you to go back to biology class, but if you understand the basics of how your skin works, you can start to understand the claims that the skincare industry is making, what works and what's totally impossible, what it does for you and what you can do for it.

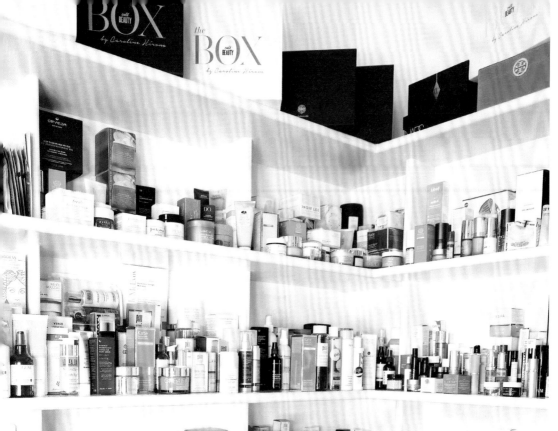
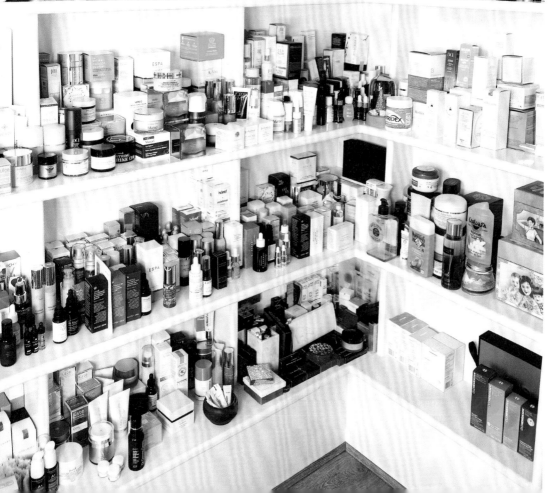

SKINCARE FOR ALL SKIN TONES

The skincare world is still way behind where it should be when it comes to showcasing, supporting and talking directly to people with darker skin tones. Ads, shades of makeup, packaging and magazines still don't feature or speak to as many non-white faces as they should, and the 'clean and wellness' industry is built on white privilege.

While the advice in this book is mostly for **all** skin tones, there are a few, but significant, differences across skin tones when it comes to taking care of your skin day to day.

THE DIFFERENCES BETWEEN DARKER AND LIGHTER SKIN TONES:

- The obvious difference is the dispersion of melanin in darker skin tones. Darker skin has more melanocytes producing melanin, which, as we've seen, is what gives your skin its colour.

- The skin barrier of darker skin can be more prone to disruption through a process of transepidermal water loss (TEWL), because of lower levels of ceramides in the stratum corneum. This means skin can feel rough and dry. When choosing moisturisers, those with darker skin may find it helpful to use products that contain natural moisturising factors (NMF), or are labelled as 'barrier repair' or 'ceramide' cream.

- As melanin offers protection from UV rays, people with darker skin tones have a natural SPF of around 13.3 compared to white skin's 3.4. This does not mean that if you have darker skin you do not need to use SPF. You do.

- Studies show that the stratum corneum is not thicker on darker skin, but it is more compact. This is good news for the elasticity and tone of darker skin.

> The skin barrier function (see Glossary) is mentioned frequently in this book. A soft, smooth-to-the-touch, plump skin is a sign of good barrier function. A compromised barrier function will present as a dull skin that feels rough and/or dry.

- A darker skin tone is more prone to hypertrophic or keloid scarring (see Glossary), where excess collagen creates a raised scar.

- Post-inflammatory hyperpigmentation (PIH) can also be an issue for people with darker skin tones. The discolouration (caused by an increase in melanin) can occur during the wound-healing process and remain after the skin has healed. When checking ingredient lists on products, look for the following to help combat this pigmentation:

  - vitamin C
  - kojic acid
  - arbutin
  - licorice extracts
  - mequinol
  - niacinamide
  - azelaic acid
  - N-acetyl glucosamine
  - hydroquinone
  - cysteamine cream
  - tretinoin

And I can't say it enough – GET YOUR SPF ON.

THE BLACK SKIN DIRECTORY

The Black Skin Directory is a brilliant resource set up by aesthetician Dija Ayodele to help people of colour in their very real struggle to find dermatologists and skincare professionals experienced in the unique demands of darker skin.

While all skin tones need a considered approach, black and darker skin tones need even more consideration due to their propensity for post-inflammatory hyperpigmentation and keloid scarring.

Dija's goal is to ensure accessibility, availability and affordability of professional skincare services for all, especially black women, who are all too often unrepresented, if not altogether ignored.

www.blackskindirectory.com

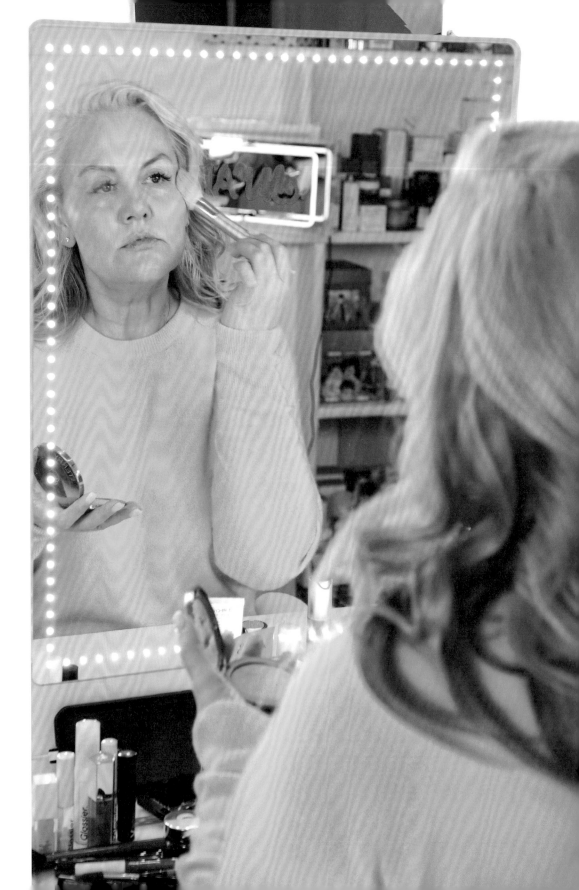

THE DIFFERENCE BETWEEN SKIN 'TYPE' AND 'CONDITION'

'Of the secrets of beauty there is but one,
and a simple one at that: make your skin work.'

— **HELENA RUBINSTEIN, 1930**

First of all, I want to clear up the difference between skin type and skin condition. The terms are often used interchangeably, but they are totally different things and you work with them in very different ways.

Your skin **type** is essentially the skin you were born with. It's what your parents gave you — it's your genes.

Most brands will try to sell you products based on your skin type when they should be targeting your skin condition. A skin **condition** generally occurs more as a result of your lifestyle or as a symptom of your skin type.

SKIN TYPE

Little did Helena Rubinstein know the effect that she would have on the skincare industry when she defined three skin types over 100 years ago. She classified skin as 'normal', 'over-moist (oily)' or 'dry', with each type determined by the level of secretions produced by the skin glands.

At its core, Rubinstein's classification is still very much relevant to today's skin 'types', which are down to your genes. However, the skincare industry now typically classifies skin into *four* types:

DRY SKIN

Usually has a lower-than-usual production of sebum, which is the oily substance your skin produces to help waterproof the skin. There may also be a lack of natural moisturising factors such as triglycerides, wax esters and squalane (see Glossary), and an impaired skin barrier. Skin will feel tight and can look dull.

OILY SKIN

Usually prone to excessive production of sebum, skin may appear shiny and thickened, and show larger pores. Blackheads and spots can be present.

NORMAL SKIN

Contains a good balance of sebum and moisturising factors. Pore size is not an issue and the skin texture is good.

COMBINATION SKIN

A mixture of skin types, and these days the most common skin type. Usually presents a slightly greasier T-zone (your forehead and nose) and dehydrated or dry cheeks.

> **NOTE:** It is entirely possible to have oily skin on the face and dry skin on the body. Your arms and legs lack sebaceous glands and therefore dry skin is far more prevalent in those areas.

It's important to identify your skin type before you invest in skincare so that the product is more likely to suit your skin. For example, a facial oil on a dry skin is lovely, but the same oil will feel heavier on an oily skin.

PORES

> My followers and clients are obsessed with pores. They say they are HUGE, then send me a picture and I can SEE NOTHING. Nobody can see your pores. The only person who can see your pores close up is your opthalmologist, facialist or aesthetician (or your partner). Your opthalmologist is looking at your eyes. Not your pores. And if your partner is **thisclosetoyou** and notices your pores, it's time for a new partner.

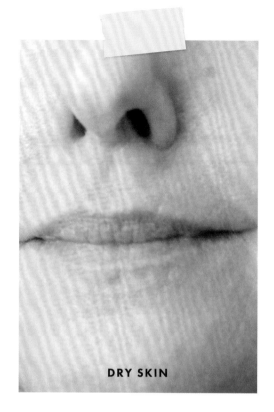

DRY SKIN

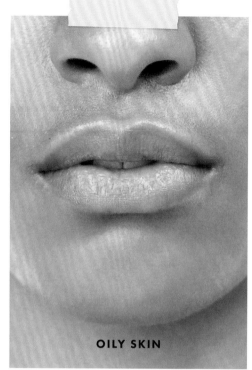

OILY SKIN

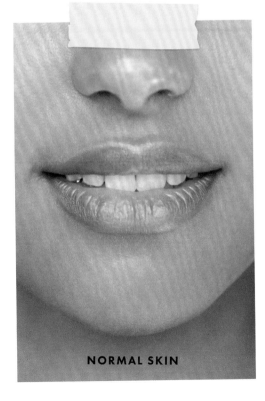

NORMAL SKIN

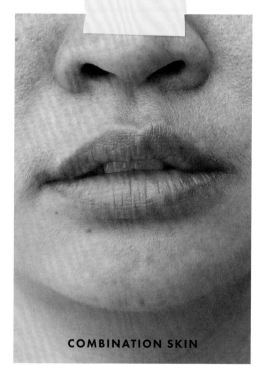

COMBINATION SKIN

SENSITIVITY

Sitting between skin 'type' and 'condition' is sensitivity. This can be genetic or lifestyle-led and it is important that you always have your skin's sensitivities at the forefront of your mind when choosing products.

SENSITIVE SKIN is increasingly common, and instances are shown to be more prevalent in women than men. Why? Men have a thicker epidermis, which seems to be a better barrier to allergens and irritants, but it is more likely that the increase is caused by the overuse of numerous products by women: as a rule, we tend to own and use more products than our male counterparts.

Dry skin will automatically be more prone to sensitivity because the barrier function (the skin's protective layer) is depleted. If your skin regularly reacts to products – for example, perhaps you've reacted to something that has caused dermatitis (inflammation of the skin) – it will likely remain sensitised for some time afterwards, and your skin will need to be treated accordingly.

TRY THESE...

- Avène Skin Recovery Cream
- Clinique Super City Block SPF40
- Curél – the entire range is for sensitivity
- Darphin Intral Daily Rescue Serum
- DeliKate® Recovery Cream
- Dermalogica UltraCalming™ Cleanser
- Jordan Samuel Skin The Aftershow Treatment Cleanser for Sensitive Skin

- Sunday Riley Juno Antioxidant + Superfood Face Oil
- Pai British Summer Time SPF30
- REN Evercalm™ Overnight Recovery Balm
- Zelens Power D Treatment Drops

SKIN CONDITION

A skin 'condition' is something that can describe either a (hopefully) temporary situation that occurs as a result of lifestyle factors, or a more long-term problem that can occur for other reasons, such as illness or inherited diseases.

'SIGNS OF AGEING' is the all-encompassing term for the skin conditions most targeted by brands, for obvious reasons. This includes everything from wrinkles to uneven skin tone, 'smile lines' to lack of elasticity in the skin.

ACNE is characterised by pustules (spots that look ready to pop, filled with pus-like fluid), blackheads and whiteheads (comedones), nodules and cysts. They are painful to the touch, and are found on the face, back ('bacne') and chest. I have found acne to be the most mentally debilitating of skin conditions in clients. Acne used to be largely found in adolescents, though it is now also extremely common in women over the age of 40. The cause is unknown and is being extensively researched by skincare brands and labs. See pages 82–87 on how to identify and treat acne.

DEHYDRATION, in my experience, is the most common skin condition and is a sign of water loss in the skin. Repair and support of the skin barrier function can aid the prevention of transepidermal water loss (TEWL). A healthy combination of fatty acids, cholesterol and ceramides, ideally in one formula (usually a serum or moisturiser), will help barrier recovery and thus prevent TEWL. Dehydrated skin absorbs moisturisers very quickly and may look dull in appearance. Products such as liquid foundations will always look uneven and patchy on a dehydrated skin.

If you suspect you have any of the conditions on the following pages, seek out a skin specialist or doctor to confirm diagnosis and suggest treatment. Where appropriate, I've suggested products that may help alleviate symptoms.

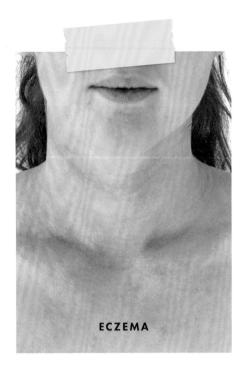

ECZEMA

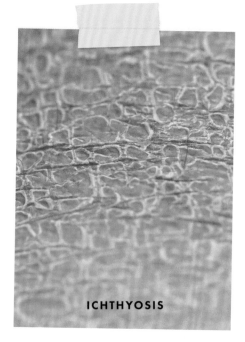

ICHTHYOSIS

ECZEMA, which can occur from birth, is itchy, inflamed and crusty skin that is sometimes sore to the touch, or swollen. Atopic eczema (atopic dermatitis) is part of a group of conditions that includes hay fever, asthma and food allergies. Sufferers generally have over-reactive inflammatory responses to environmental factors and products such as detergents, and it tends to run in families. If you suffer from eczema, you will gain some immediate relief from using rich moisturisers such as those listed below.

TRY THESE...

- Avène
- Diprobase®
- Eucerin
- Mother Dirt AO+ Mist
- Weleda Skin Food

ICHTHYOSIS is the continual scaling of the skin (build-up of skin cells). It can occur on any area of the body and presents as extremely dry, cracked skin. There are many forms of ichthyosis, the most common being the inherited ichthyosis vulgaris. Sufferers of this type of ichthyosis are shown to have a gene defect in filaggrin, a protein in the skin that impairs the formation of a healthy skin barrier and the natural moisturising factors (NMF) that are key to keeping the skin hydrated. Seek out a skin specialist or doctor to confirm diagnosis and suggest treatment.

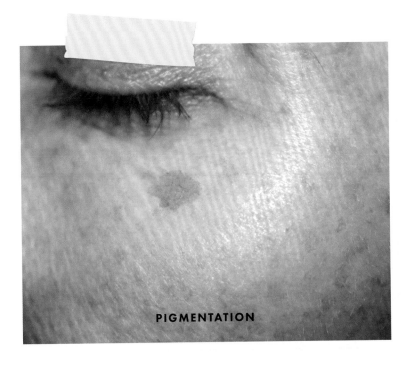

PIGMENTATION

PIGMENTATION issues arise either through age, sun exposure, hormonal changes or physical damage to the skin and are usually caused by a combination of factors. Pigmentation issues include melasma (see page 103) – also called chloasma – and PIH (post-inflammatory hyperpigmentation) – or PIPA (post-inflammatory pigment alteration) – which is extremely common in darker skin tones and usually happens after an injury to the skin. If you have pigmentation issues of any kind, you need to use a high SPF daily and invest in serums that target this condition.

TRY THESE...

- Dermalogica Powerbright Dark Spot Serum

- Murad Rapid Age Spot Correcting Serum

- NIOD RE:Pigment

- The Ordinary Alpha Arbutin 2% + HA or Niacinamide 10% + Zinc 1%

KERATOSIS PILARIS (aka 'chicken skin') is thought to be associated with, or in the same family as, eczema and ichthyosis. It presents as bumps most commonly found at the top of your arms and thighs, giving the appearance of goose bumps. 'Pilaris' (from the Latin for 'hair'), and 'keratosis' (too much keratin), simply means that you have extra keratin accumulating in your hair follicles. It is harmless, and not contagious, but it can be annoying for the sufferer. You can help remedy it by body brushing and using dedicated acid-based moisturisers on the area. My readers have found that taking their acid-soaked cotton pad over the areas of keratosis pilaris on a daily basis after using it on their face helped with the 'chicken skin' on their arms.

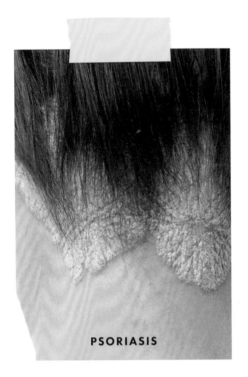

PSORIASIS

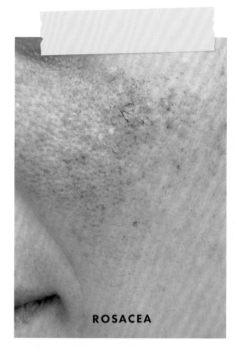

ROSACEA

PSORIASIS is an autoimmune inflammatory disease that presents with dry, red, itchy and scaly skin in patches, predominantly on the elbows, knees, lower back and scalp. Most skin cells take 3–4 weeks to move up through the layers of the skin. In psoriasis, that process takes 3–7 days, leading to the cells stacking on top of each other and giving a white, silverish effect to the skin's surface. You would be hard pushed to find an over-the-counter product that will fix psoriasis. Stick with the prescription goods.

ROSACEA is a much-recognised auto-inflammatory skin condition that has numerous symptoms and different levels of diagnosis. Symptoms can be as mild as flushing, and as intense as swelling, burning and stinging. It tends to be episodic, flaring up when aggravated, and will in all likelihood make you sun-sensitive. It can be triggered by alcohol consumption, extreme temperatures, stress, exercise and the consumption of spicy foods. Treatment for rosacea is unique to the individual, but using anti-inflammatories such as over-the-counter azelaic acid, along with SPF, is key. If you have rosacea you may prefer a mineral SPF, as they are usually tolerated better than chemical blockers. Early diagnosis is shown to help slow down progression. If you're a long-term rosacea sufferer, you should be under a clinician's care. OTC (Over the Counter) products may help relieve the symptoms of subtype 1. All the other types require the attention of a doctor, and prescriptions.

Rosacea is categorised medically by four subtypes (patients may suffer with more than one type):

Subtype 1: Erythematotelangiectatic rosacea. Sufferers may present with facial flushing, swelling and telangiectasia (broken capillaries/spider veins).

Subtype 2: Papulopustular rosacea. Sometimes misdiagnosed as acne, this is 'classic rosacea' and typically presents with persistent redness across the central panel of the face and occasional papules and pustules.

Subtype 3: Phymatous rosacea. Most commonly seen in older men, this affects the nasal area and can also present on the chin and cheeks. Skin will appear thickened and uneven, with a rough surface. It can be treated with lasers, isotretinoin and, in extreme cases, surgery.

Subtype 4: Ocular rosacea. Sometimes going undiagnosed for many years, this is literally rosacea around the eye area and can present as stinging, burning and watering of the eyes along with common occurrences of blepharitis and conjunctivitis.

TRY THESE...

- Ecooking™ Sunscreen SPF30
- Elizabeth Arden Advanced Ceramide Capsules Daily Youth Restoring Serum
- Paula's Choice 10% Azelaic Acid Booster
- Paula's Choice Clinical Ceramide-Enriched Moisturiser
- Sunday Riley ICE Ceramide Moisturizing Cream
- The Ordinary Azelaic Acid Suspension 10%

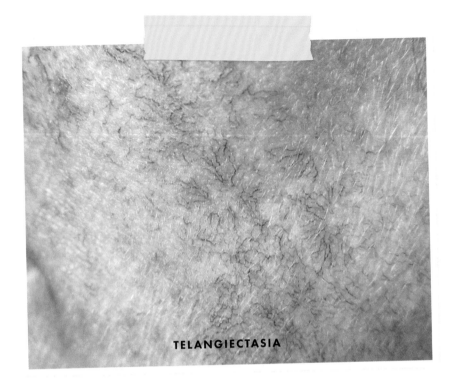

TELANGIECTASIA

Couperose sits in the rosacea family and is caused by small blood vessels on the cheeks, nose, forehead or chin expanding and losing their elasticity. It generally causes permanent redness and can be accompanied by a feeling of heat, burning or tingling. Bear in mind it's exacerbated by heat.

TELANGIECTASIA is more commonly known as broken capillaries. You may be more prone to these if your parents have them. They are extremely common and appear more noticeable in paler skins. It is a common condition in skins with rosacea.

VITILIGO is a chronic condition that can start at birth and usually presents before adulthood. People with vitiligo have the same number of melanocytes (the cells that decide your skin tone) as a person without, but the melanocytes are inactive, leading to patches of paler/pinker skin. Vitiligo affects both men and women equally, but is more noticeable in people of colour. It is considered an autoimmune condition as the body's immune system appears to reject its own cells (in this case, melanocytes). Seek out a skin specialist or doctor to confirm diagnois and suggest treatment.

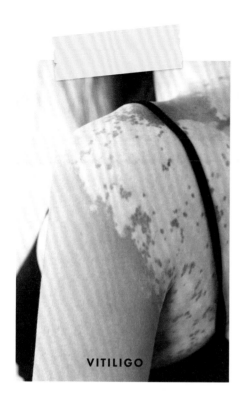

VITILIGO

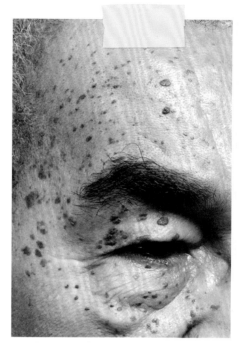

DERMATOSIS PAPULOSA NIGRA

People with darker skin tones are found to be more prone to these conditions:

PROBLEMATIC INGROWN HAIRS, known as *pseudofolliculitis* (and *pseudofolliculitis barbae* for the beard area), or more commonly as 'razor bumps' or 'shaving bumps'. This inflammation of the hair follicles and the surrounding area is due to hair being trapped in the follicle. It is caused when fragile Afro hair is removed, most commonly by shaving, and retreats in on itself due to its helix-like shape.

DERMATOSIS PAPULOSA NIGRA (DPN). This affects black skin more than any other skin tone. It presents as small, benign skin lesions that can clump together on the skin, forming the appearance of bigger patches. They are thought to be genetic and are not harmful, although people with DPN may seek to get them removed. I would urge you to research all medical options and only consider treatment with doctors fully versed in the possible known side effects of treatment on darker skin tones, such as scarring, postoperative hyper/hypo skin pigmentation and the potential for keloid scarring. Surgical removal options include curettage (scraping), cryotherapy and laser therapy.

IS YOUR SKIN DRY OR DEHYDRATED (OR BOTH)?

Dry skins and dehydrated skins can have very similar characteristics, but different underlying causes, and interestingly blur the line between skin type and skin condition.

DRY SKIN

Dry skin is normally a skin type *but* it *can* also be a temporary skin condition. It is caused by lack of oil in the skin. Characteristics of dry skin include:

- Small pores
- Skin feels 'tight'
- Skin may be flaky
- Milia, blackheads and spots may be present
- Skin looks dull
- Skin is not plump
- Skin doesn't absorb products easily
- Skin is easily irritated and more likely to suffer reactions to products
- Skin is aggravated by poor skincare

DEHYDRATED SKIN

A skin condition such as dehydration can affect any skin type, including dry and oily skin. It is caused by lack of water in the skin (not lack of water taken orally!). Characteristics of dehydrated skin include:

- Pores can be large or small
- Skin feels 'tight' and dry, although confusingly, in the case of oily skin, it can still look shiny and have breakouts
- Skin absorbs moisturisers really quickly
- Blackheads and spots are still visible
- Makeup disappears (and goes patchy) throughout the day as the skin is absorbing any water in your foundation
- Skin looks 'ashen'
- A possibility of suffering from headaches

In normal circumstances, your hydrolipidic film (on the surface of the skin) acts as a regulator and barrier – retaining moisture and protecting your skin against germs. If, for whatever reason, that film's effectiveness is affected, the moisture in the epidermis evaporates too quickly and the normal, healthy state of the skin is compromised.

The reality is that most of us at one time or another have dehydrated skin. Any and all of the following can cause dehydration:

ENVIRONMENT: Wind, cold air, dry air, too much sun, air conditioning, central heating

HYDRATION: Consuming alcohol and caffeine, not eating enough water-heavy foods or not drinking enough water

LIFESTYLE: Stress, poor skincare routine, using the wrong products, medication (including birth control) or smoking

GENETICS: Monthly cycle, pregnancy or hormones

A WORD ON SUPPLEMENTS

Although Omega oils found in either flax or fish oil supplements may help both dry and dehydrated skins, you need to be using them for at least 3 months before you'll see the benefits on your skin.

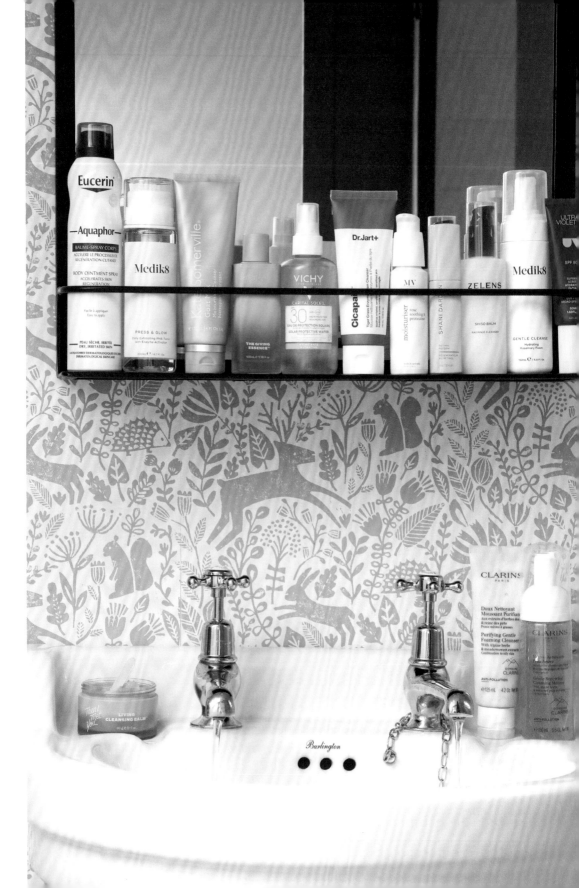

It is quite common to have skin that is both dry and dehydrated, but if the definitions on the previous pages have helped you ascertain that your skin is either dry or dehydrated (or both), these dos and don'ts might help:

- **Do** upgrade your moisturiser to one suitable for dry skin if you recognise the signs – go for products using the words 'nourishing'.

- **Do** change your moisturiser to one labelled 'hydra' or 'hydrating' if you suspect you are dehydrated.

- **Do** use balms, oils and serums for dry skin.

- **Do** use milks, specified oils and treatments for dehydrated skin.

- **Do not** use products that are too harsh or too stripping.

- **Steer clear of harsh foaming products** – keep the bubbles for your dishes.

- Whether your skin is dry or dehydrated, adding a little hyaluronic acid (see Glossary) to your routine won't hurt.

TRY THESE...

- Bioderma Hydrabio Crème
- Chanticaille Pure Rosewater
- Darphin Rose Aromatic Care
- Dr.Jart+™ Cicapair™ Tiger Grass Calming Mist
- Hada Labo Tokyo™– range is made for dehydrated skins
- Murad Hydro-Dynamic Quenching Essence
- Neutrogena Hydro Boost Water Gel Moisturiser
- NIOD Multi-Molecular Hyaluronic Complex MMCH2
- Weleda Skin Food

HUNGOVER, PARCHED OR WEATHER-WORN SKIN

The three main culprits of dehydrated, parched and dry skin are over-indulgence in alcohol, salt and sugar.

The effects these have on the skin are similar to those experienced by many teachers, nurses and doctors who work in dry, warm, germ-festering classrooms and insanely hot hospitals. If you've overdosed on 'All I Want for Christmas Is You', you live somewhere with four seasons, or your professional environment is taking its toll, and you've noticed that your skin is not itself and/or that your lips are so dry that they feel like they may split, tackling these potential causes may help...

ALCOHOL

There are no two ways about it: booze is dreadful for your skin. It dehydrates you to the point of raisin-like status, and if you are slack in your skin-product usage because of the effects of alcohol, it will only get worse. If you are prone to reddening (see rosacea, pages 118–119), alcohol will give you a helping hand to the point where you could easily understudy for Rudolph.

SALT

Puffy/bloated and dehydrated? Those heavy dinners, gravy and salty snacks may have taken hold. And, if your indulgences are of the sweeter nature, blame...

SUGAR

This is the Devil for your skin and your internal organs. That's basically all. You may as well take a hammer and chisel to your collagen. Sugar causes glycation (see Glossary), which in turn makes it much harder for your skin to produce healthy collagen. It literally puts a spanner in the works.

Take all three of these culprits together and you may look in the mirror with some concern. Fear not. It's easily fixed: drink water like it's going out of fashion. First thing, on the hour every hour, and before bed (if you don't already). Rehydrate yourself.

WHAT IF YOUR WORKPLACE IS NOT HELPING YOUR SKIN?

I know this is particularly difficult for teachers. Do what you can, when you get a break. Nurses: keep a water bottle on your station and keep it filled.

Drinking water will give you clarity of mind and help prevent headaches, but how much water you drink sadly has little effect on the hydration levels of your skin. It won't hurt, but it's not the cure.

Follow my tips on a skincare routine for dry and/or dehydrated skin on pages 76–79.

ACNE

Acne is a skin condition that presents typically as a combination of blackheads, whiteheads and spots or cysts on the face and neck (and sometimes the back and chest). It can be severe and distressing, and the psychological effects it can have on sufferers should not be ignored.

We tend to associate acne with puberty and teens, but when I turned 40, **out of nowhere** I experienced adult-onset acne, along with food allergies. And it has become increasingly obvious to me that the same is happening to a lot of women. I had near-perfect skin for 40 years and then, suddenly, a face full of red, angry cysts. My doctor put me straight on antibiotics and I, in my desperation, took them unquestioningly.

Once I realised that the acne was more than likely hormonal, and that the antibiotics were doing me no favours, I decided to fix it myself: I stopped taking the antibiotics, adjusted my diet (I'm not going to tell you what I did and didn't eat, because I'm not a dietician) and changed my skincare. Where I'd previously used heavier moisturising products, I switched to more hyaluronic acid serums and oil-free moisturisers and this did the trick. The reason I am giving you so much background is because you need to give the same care to your skin.

There is **no magical 'cure'** for acne. There are different types, yes, but no one-dose-fits-all cure. Do read the below, but bear in mind that acne is different for everyone. You may have one type – or three types. You need to know your whole 'system' – skin, body and state of mind – to see results.

TYPES OF ACNE

HORMONAL ACNE: can occur if you're just starting periods, just finishing periods, experiencing perimenopause or menopause. Raging androgen in boys can also cause over-production of oil, slow shedding of dead skin cells, which all create the perfect breeding ground for acne.

SENSITIVITY-RELATED ACNE: can be related to allergies, an adverse reaction to a product, or reactions to foods (such as shellfish) or your environment.

"
YOU NEED TO KNOW YOUR SKIN, YOUR BODY AND YOUR STATE OF MIND INSIDE OUT TO TRULY SEE RESULTS

"

The two key cuplrits are **bacteria** and **inflammation**.

Propionibacterium acnes is the bacteria that gives our friend acne its name. All it needs is the perfect environment in order to spread.

Inflammation can be caused by illness, foods or stress – a system fighting illness is inflamed. Add medication and you are doubling your potential problems. Foods can cause inflammation (especially food allergies) and stress always causes inflammation – these are all breeding grounds for acne.

Looking at the above you may see where your skin fits in, and why antibiotics just will not work for some people (the exception is when they are prescribed as part of a full regimen from a dermatologist).

A WORD ON ANTIBIOTICS

Antibiotics can save your life. Literally. I'm not bashing the drugs. I'm bashing the over-prescribing of them by some doctors, specifically GPs (not dermatologists), who should know better. If you are taking antibiotics for a skin problem and they haven't 'done anything' – something I hear a lot – consider stopping taking them (in line with your practitioner's advice). They are bad for your digestive system and make you massively susceptible to severe sun damage. They wreak havoc on your tooth enamel, too, and can make you resistant to antibiotic usage for severe infections.

Instead of referring you to a specialist dermatologist, some doctors insist on giving out repeat prescriptions for skins that are not responding to them because they don't know any better. If your acne is really bad, ask for a referral to a hospital consultant or specialist unit. You may not get a referral unless it is visibly bad: a few hormonal spots once a month, requiring you to break out the heavy-duty concealer, is not on a par with the suffering of people with the severest cases. Ask for that referral if you need it, or pay to see a dermatologist. Invest in your skin.

MYTHS AND OLD WIVES' TALES

It seems that once something has been said in a glossy mag or seen on TV (or both) it becomes The Law. Sad but true. And this is not helpful to those of us with real problems that we want to fix. Here are a few untruths out there:

- **Acne is caused by dirty skin.** Not true. There is a massive difference between bacteria and dirt. Over-washing your face destroys the acid mantle that protects your skin (the very fine acidic film on the surface of the skin that is your first line of defence against bacteria and viruses), creates an alkaline environment and makes your acne worse and your skin a dry, dull, sore breeding ground. Having said that, I highly recommend that you regularly change your pillowcases (at least once a week).

- **You can 'dry up' spots.** Not true. A spot is a mixture of oil, inflammation, bacteria and dead skin cells. There's no water in that list. All you are doing is drying the surrounding area in the hope that it will make the spot look smaller. What it actually does is put the spot on its own 'look at ME' platform.

- **You can use toothpaste or nappy/diaper cream to spot-treat acne.** A one-off spot may have its redness taken down – temporarily – by applying one of these, but they won't get rid of acne. If acne could be fixed by what you're using on your teeth or your baby's backside, all of our problems would be solved. Dude. **Stop putting toothpaste and bum cream on your face**.

THINGS THAT MAY HELP

Thanks to my friends, clients and readers of my blog, I've created a list of things that have helped some people with their acne over the years. It is not definitive, but rather a list of suggestions. They may not work for you or they may work brilliantly – unfortunately, there is no perfect solution.

- **Avoid too much alcohol in products.** A 'tingle' is okay, but 'burning' is not. Products where the main ingredient listed is alcohol will dry out the surface of your skin, destroy the acid mantle and make the perfect breeding ground for bacteria. However, alcohol in acids is the exception: alcohol is sometimes a necessary evil for suspending things like glycolic acid in a solution where they would normally not work as well.

- **Do not completely strip your skin of oil and moisture.** An acneic skin that sticks solely to traditional 'foaming' cleansers and oil-free products is nearly always – always – reddened with inflammation and sensitivity. Alkaline soaps and some foaming washes that contain SLS will contribute to the breakdown of the acid mantle of your skin and take your skin to the wrong end of the acid/alkaline scale. It's called acid mantle for a reason. Remember litmus paper from science classes? Alkaline skin is the perfect breeding ground for bacteria.

- **Do not pick red cysts.** A whitehead can be popped in the correct manner (see pages 232–235).

> A cyst is going nowhere and will always, always prevail if you battle it. And then it will scar, just to teach you who is boss.

- **Avoid moisturisers made with good-quality, heavy shea butter.** Yes, it's natural, but it's harder than most oils for the skin to break down and thus tends to clogs pores and give you nice whiteheads. Buy moisturisers with water as the main ingredient for daytime use. You can use appropriate oils and balms at night.

- **Treat your skin gently and with respect.** You know what I mean. Abusing it with harsh products and getting angry with it as if it's a different person will make it worse. Your skin belongs to you. Do not try to disown it when it needs you.

- **Cleanse with good-quality oils and balm cleansers.** There is absolutely no reason to avoid oil when you have acne. Avoid mineral oil, yes, but good, light, plant-derived oils do not clog pores; they nourish the skin you are now pledging to take care of, and they do not cause breakouts.

- **Use topical exfoliants.** Using acids topically will help tackle blocked pores, remove dead skin cells, trapped hair follicles and reduce your acid mantle to the lower end of the scale – usually around a 3 or 4 – which is, in layman's terms, strengthening your first line of defence to the acne. Use glycolic, lactic or salicylic acid (see pages 122–129 for more information on acids).

- **You can use products containing benzoyl peroxide or sulphur,** found in spot treatments, to topically treat bad acne spots. It can penetrate the pore and kill off the bacteria specific to acne, but I prefer to use the acids I mention in the step above. A word of warning: both are extremely drying to the skin in high percentages. Go easy.

- **Hydrate your skin and consider that it might need facial oil in places.** You can have acne in some areas and be really dry or dehydrated in others.

- **Consider supplementation.** Probiotics are a must, especially if you are on antibiotics. Your skin is the first part of your body that will indicate if there's something going wrong in the gut. Keep your stomach and intestines as strong as possible. Go for the highest dosage of probiotics you can find and be aware that they have a short shelf life and may not be as effective as the label states. As always, speak to your consultant before supplementing.

Stress is the key to most flare-ups, whether they are acne, rosacea or eczema. Practise relaxation. And not in some hippy-dippy way. Seriously. See the bigger picture. Chill.

TRY THESE...

- Clarins UV Plus Anti-Pollution SPF50 Rose
- Dermatica – online prescription service
- Kate Somerville Oil-Free Moisturiser
- La Roche-Posay Effaclar H Moisturiser
- May Lindstrom The Problem Solver
- Paula's Choice Clear Regular Strength 2% BHA Exfoliant
- Paula's Choice Skin Balancing Moisturiser SPF30

- REN Clean Skincare ClearCalm Non-Drying Spot Treatment
- Renée Rouleau Anti Bump Solution
- Skin + Me – online prescription service
- Skingredients Sally Cleanse
- Summer Fridays Cloud Dew Oil-Free Gel Cream Moisturizer
- Sunday Riley Ceramic Slip Cleanser
- ZitSticka GOO GETTER™ Surface Zit Hydrocolloid Patch

!?#

SKIN PURGING

Your skin should not 'purge' (heavily break out) when using over-the-counter (OTC) acne products. Prescription-strength products given to you by a dermatologist for acne, for example, can cause purging, but these are drugs and the purging will happen under the care of a medical professional. For example, if you are put on a medical regimen to tackle acne, you may well purge for a good few weeks, even a couple of months (some patients find this the most trying part of a new routine, but eventually it is worth it).

However, if you start using a new OTC product and suddenly have a face full of spots, redness or swelling, it is likely that the product (or machine) is not for you. However, strong OTC retinoids (vitamin A treatments) can cause purging, and in that case, I would recommend down-scaling to a milder one until your skin adjusts. There may be a risk of slight exacerbation of spots if you are acneic and suddenly use a product high in salicylic acid, for example, but that should not last for weeks on end.

I often come across products that claim, 'This may make your skin purge for a while, but then it will be GREAT!' The reality is probably closer to 'This may give you a face full of spots, either because the ingredients are comedogenic (block pores), or your skin does not like some of the ingredients'. The odd whitehead (i.e. a proper, traditional spot) appearing after using a new product is no big deal.

An angry red face with a mixture of swollen, won't-come-to-a-head spots, cysts, whiteheads and blackheads is not 'purging'. It's your skin begging you to stop whatever it is you are doing. Listen to it.

Personally, even if my skin was bubbling under the surface like a dormant volcano, I'd rather treat it gently. I do not want to use something that makes it erupt. Hey ho, that's just moi.

MASKNE

Since *Skincare* was first published, the world has been turned on its head by Covid-19. We suddenly all had to get used to wearing masks in public spaces. The effect on our skin from this is two-fold: presenting as either acne breakouts or red, irritated skin, especially in medical staff who are wearing full PPE (personal protective equipment) for extended periods of time.

The main thing to remember is that, on this occasion, the problems with your skin are circumstantial. This isn't genetics, it's literally happening as a result of a situation that you cannot control.

Masks, as crucial as they are, cause the perfect breeding ground for bacteria: it's dark, damp and warm in there. It's essentially a holiday camp for germs.

The other main antagonist here is stress.

And who isn't stressed when there is a global pandemic happening? Stress causes your cortisol levels to rise, which in turn causes your body to crank up oil production, leading to spots/more spots/irritation.

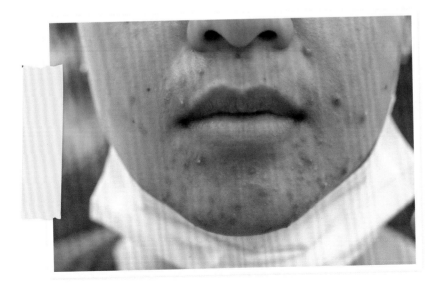

SO, WHAT CAN YOU DO?

There are some general guidelines to follow to prevent breakouts of 'maskne', namely:

- Use products aimed at a sensitive skin.
- Choose fragrance free where possible.
- Avoid wearing makeup/foundation under your mask if you can. Emphasise your eyes instead!
- Pick products, especially moisturisers, that contain ceramides to help keep your skin barrier intact. Most suitable products will mention 'skin barrier repair' in their descriptions or titles.

IF WEARING MASKS HAS GIVEN YOU A BAD BREAKOUT:

- Wash your face with a benzoyl peroxide-containing cleanser 2–3 x a week.
- Exfoliate regularly with either a salicylic or glycolic acid.
- Stop using heavy, rich moisturisers.
- Use lightweight lotions or serums that are based around glycerin.
- Avoid tretinoin (prescription vitamin A) and use over the counter retinols instead. They are more gentle.

IF YOUR SKIN IS RED, BRUISED OR SENSITISED:

- Niacinamide should help to reduce redness and inflammation.
- Hyaluronic acid is good for speeding up skin healing.
- Use gentle cleansers that you can splash off without needing a washcloth/flannel that could cause more irritation.
- If your skin is really sore and irritated, try some occlusives such as Vaseline or nappy/diaper cream. This is probably the only time you'll hear me say this so enjoy it:

Apply a little petroleum jelly/nappy cream around your mouth/sides of your nostrils or across the bridge of your nose, wherever you have the irritation. Remember to keep it away from the edges of the mask or you risk breaking the seal of your mask.

66

THIS IS PROBABLY THE ONLY TIME YOU'LL HEAR ME SAY THIS SO ENJOY IT

99

SKINCARE MYTH

HAVING SPOTS MEANS YOU HAVE ACNE OR OILY/COMBINATION SKIN

Most of the people I see have normal, dehydrated or sensitive skin with occasional spots. This is very different to acne. There are two vicious circles you can get into that can lead to occasional spots.

VICIOUS CIRCLE ONE

You had acne as a teenager and are now in your 20s, 30s or 40s+ and continue to treat your skin as if it is acneic. In fact, your skin moved on when you were 19 or 20. Underneath that redness and sensitivity is actually normal skin. The redness and sensitivity have been caused by years of using products for oily/combination skin that dry it out and 'mattify' it (*cries*), causing it to over-produce oil, give you angry red spots, burning cheeks and lead you to think that you are still an oily/combo skin and that your skin hates you. And usually this makes you hate your skin and despair.

VICIOUS CIRCLE TWO

You once had a few breakouts and you went to a beauty counter or had a facial where you were told you had oily/combination skin because your sales assistant or therapist's training led them to believe spots = acne = oily/combination = foaming = mattifying.

Your skin was actually pretty normal. Now it's oily because it's dried out and is desperately trying to replenish itself, so your skin is oily by midday or 3pm and you keep thinking that you have an 'oily' skin. You therefore think you are doing everything wrong and your skin hates you. And usually this vicious circle will also make you hate your skin and despair.

I'm not suggesting that occasional spots are not a serious condition and mentally taxing, I'm simply suggesting that we overuse the word 'acne' across the industry and do not train our people well enough to detect the difference between acne and hormonal breakouts, food intolerance spots, product reactions or other reactions. Most people I see with breakouts have a normal, slightly dehydrated or sensitised skin with spots. That is very different to acne. It can happen to anyone, at any time, for any reason.

So please, please, the next time you have breakouts – even if they are multiple or in different areas of the face, and at different times of the month – they are spots. Do not treat your entire face as if you have acne/combination skin. Think about what it could be. Have you done anything differently? Have you ever had intolerance tests for food groups? Is your period due? Have you been on a three-day bender? Are you using a sodium lauryl sulphate (SLS) shampoo in the shower and letting it run all over your face?

Treat the spots by taking care of the skin. Your skin is not your enemy – do not treat it like it is. Spots and acne are two very different things.

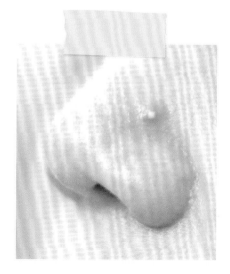

SPOTS

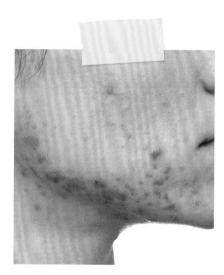

ACNE

PERIORAL DERMATITIS

(aka 'those red annoying spots that won't go away')

- You've had spots, redness, flakiness or something that looks like (but isn't) eczema or acne, for ages, in one place around your mouth, nose or eyes. The spots are not particularly big, they don't seem to want to LEAVE and sometimes they appear to multiply.

- You have clusters of spots, redness or flaking around your nose or mouth that laugh at you and say, 'nice try!' when you apply spot treatment.

- Sometimes the spots sting or burn.

- Sometimes the spots flake over and literally peel off.

- Sometimes the spots disappear altogether and give you a sense of satisfaction, then POP BACK UP AS IF LIKE MAGIC.

- The thought of using something harsh such as an exfoliating acid on the area makes you feel a tad faint.

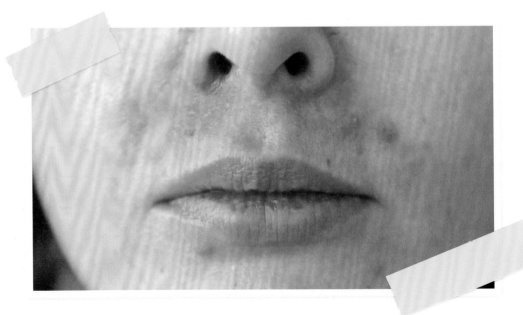

Does this sound familiar? You may have perioral dermatitis (or periorificial dermatitis if it's around your eyes). Do not panic or worry. It's very common and easily fixed. If you ignore it, however, it can spread.

While it occurs predominantly in women aged 20–45, giving it a possible hormonal factor, men and children can also be affected. The causes are multiple, and the triggers can be a combination of things:

- A reaction to some cosmetic products
- A reaction to steroid creams (often referred to as steroid rosacea)
- Strong winds / UV light (think joggers and chapped skin)
- Hormonal contraception
- Dribbling in your sleep
- Fluoride in toothpaste
- Sodium lauryl sulphate (SLS) in toothpaste and cleansers

The parts of the face affected are near areas that are warm, dark and wet – the perfect combination for bacterial growth.

It's easy to treat. If it is a recurring problem, visit your doctor. You will be prescribed a topical cream, or oral antibiotics if it's really severe. Avoid applying active ingredients to the area until it subsides. Good, plain nourishing oils such as jojoba – or one that contains vitamin D – will help to stop the itchiness and remedy the dryness. **The biggest single difference for me personally was using toothpaste that did not contain any SLS. I avoid it completely now.**

MILIA

Stubborn, unsightly and annoyingly hard to get rid of, milia are found in people of all ages. Babies, kids and adults can all be affected. All races and genders. Milia do not discriminate. They generally affect the thin skin around the eyes and upper parts of the cheeks in adults, and are basically a mini cyst: a cyst full of keratin. We like keratin — we need it. It's what gives our skin, hair and nails structure. You just don't want it trapped under your skin and trying to get out.

The important things to remember are:
- They're NOT spots
- They have nothing to do with your pores — milia are under your epidermis
- They're not harmful
- They're not infectious
- They're not caused by germs or bacteria
- You can't get rid of them by taking an antibiotic or the contraceptive pill

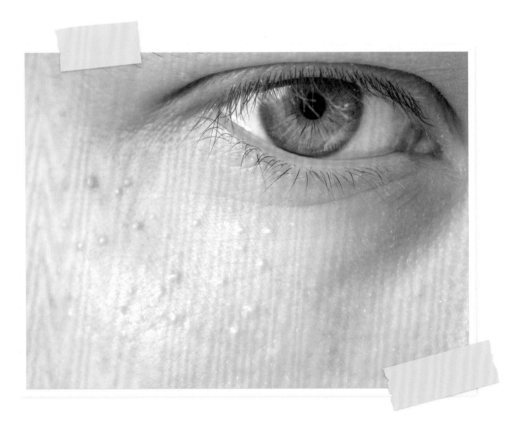

If you have a lot of them – and if your family also suffer with them – it's likely you're genetically predisposed to them. If you just get the odd one here and there you probably just need to up the ante on your skincare routine.

HOW TO GET RID OF LARGER MILIA

First of all, **don't bother trying to pick at milia**. You're setting yourself up for a whole heap of trouble. Essentially what this will do is pick a hole in your skin.

- **Get a professional to remove them.** Phone your nearest salon. Ask them specifically if they remove milia. Double check. Say, 'Do you *physically* remove milia?' We're talking manually – no microdermabrasion, no laser – just your therapist, her steady hand and a suitable needle. If they hesitate, don't go. You do not want someone who's not confident and well-trained poking around your eye area with a needle. Few salons offer the service – in some districts you're not allowed to 'pierce the skin' in a salon (this is down to old legislation relating to sex clubs in city centres, not facials).

- **Go see a dermatologist** – let them deal with them.

HOW TO HELP SHIFT SMALLER MILIA

Well, to start with, get into a routine every day that makes your skin work for itself.

- **Keep your skin well cleansed,** using flannels and warm water (see pages 110–116).

- **Exfoliate every day** (gently – don't go tearing at your skin or the area of milia) and do not – repeat after me – DO NOT use any of those apricot scrubs you can get in the chemist. EVER. END OF.

- **Alternate between a topical acid toner and a hydrating toner/ essence** (a really runny serum). Toners or toning lotions are essential for controlling milia. The acid toner – used on the area affected by the milia only – will help shift the surface layers of the skin quicker, the hydrating one will ensure you don't dry your face out at the same time. It takes 2 seconds. Use the acid toner first, the hydrating toner second.

- **Keep the milia moisturised.**

- You may like to **use a clay mask** occasionally, in the privacy of your own home. Just do your nightly cleanse, whack it on the area and have dinner/ watch telly/whatever – remove, tone, moisturise.

You should find that some of the smaller milia shift themselves doing this. Also, follow these general guidelines:

Do not pick at the milia with needles – if you don't know what you're doing you'll scar your face.

Do use a topical acid on the area, exfoliate regularly, moisturise normally, and use good-quality clay masks on the area regularly. If you wish, get the milia removed safely by a professional.

"
DO NOT COMPLAIN ABOUT TIME TAKEN TO TAKE CARE OF YOUR FACE.
IT'S YOUR *FACE*
"

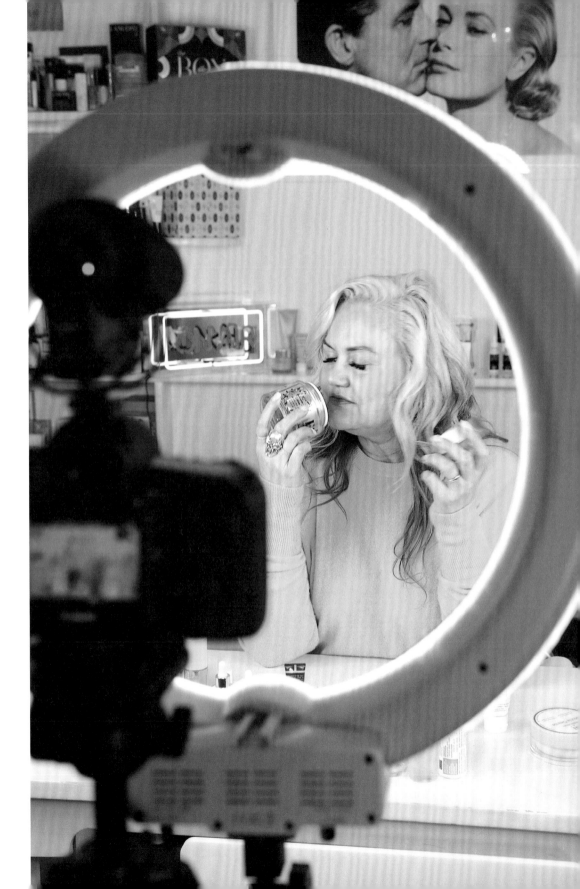

HOW TO TREAT YOUR SKIN

Now that you know a bit more about how your skin works, how do you treat it?

Very few of us have what could be termed 'normal skin', which is why I find it odd that there's a skin type called 'normal'.

For most of us, there are multiple issues to contend with: pigmentation, rosacea, dry skin, oily skin, combination skin, sensitive skin, dehydrated skin – you name it, you probably have at least one of them.

But, what if you have **more than one?** What if you have three skin issues? Or four?

'Normal skin' is far from the norm for most people. It's not uncommon, for example, to see a dehydrated, hyper-pigmented, sensitive, ageing skin with hormonal breakouts. Dr Leslie Baumann gave us her 16 skin types years ago, and she was spot on, although I think there are even more than that. Start by treating your skin according to the potential your issue has to cause pain and/or long-lasting damage, such as scarring or broken capillaries.

#1
First, take care of sensitivity or rosacea. Inflammation will exacerbate the other issues. For example, if you have rosacea and acne and use a traditional foaming acne 'wash', your cheeks will scream at you. That's not good. That's not what you need or want for your face.

Sensitivity is King. Best product choice: moisturiser or a fragrance-free facial oil designed for sensitive skin.

#2
Tackle dehydration. Dehydrated skin drinks anything you put on it, but you have to hydrate it repeatedly: your anti-ageing serums end up just filling a gap in your skin rather than actually doing their job.

If you are dehydrated, you can leave the house in the morning with perfectly hydrated, bouncy skin and it will be dehydrated to the point of it showing on facial machinery by mid-morning. No matter what you do, what you use, how old you are, or your lifestyle, you can be dehydrated just by waking up. You need to treat the dehydration.

Best product choice: those in the toning phase – use both acid and spritz, followed by serum. Use acid on cotton pads to gently strip back the skin and then spritz with a mist containing hyaluronic acid, glycerin (or both) and follow with hyaluronic acid serum. None of these products should irritate any of the other issues.

#3   **Now you can start to be more general.** As long as you are keeping your redness under control and your skin hydrated, you can tackle anything. Here are the best product choices for the following skin types or conditions:

DRY SKIN: use facial oils and oil in products including balm cleansers – no foam, ever. Dryness frequently overlaps with dehydration. If your skin is both dry and dehydrated, treat both issues simultaneously, and if you are unsure which you are, read pages 76–79.

AGEING SKIN: use targeted serums; think retinoids and peptides.

PIGMENTED SKIN: use dedicated serums for pigmentation, retinoids and SPF (I'm not suggesting you don't use SPF under normal circumstances; it's just the priority if you scar easily, get sun spots etc.).

OILY SKIN: use acid toners and a suitable serum and moisturiser. Do not over-embrace oil-free and harsh, stripping, foaming products.

ACNE: the acid toning phase is key, as is your moisturiser. Please, please think carefully about how you will go about replenishing the oils in your skin if you use an oil-free moisturiser. If you want to try to keep your oil under control by mid-afternoon, use an oil-free moisturiser if you want to, but use a facial oil dedicated for acne/combination skin underneath it. I promise, a drop or two can make all the difference. We're ahead of the game now and the skincare market has plenty.

The old 'foam wash, alcohol-laden strip-tone, oil-free moisturiser' routine is dead and buried. Or should be.

And, finally, a special mention to the sufferers of melasma – or chloasma, as it may be called by your midwife if you're pregnant.

Melasma and pigmentation are different things:

PIGMENTATION can be caused by sun damage, acne scarring, picking spots or inflammation, and can normally be treated with topical products – glycolic, kojic and azaleic acids, retinoids and liquorice, for example – with some success.

Best product choices: peels, and targeted serums containing those ingredients and SPF.

MELASMA can be *triggered* by the same things that cause pigmentation but is also linked to hormones (hence the link to pregnancy, the contraceptive pill and perimenopausal women) and illnesses such as Addison's disease, lupus and coeliac disease. Female sufferers outnumber male nine to one. It's basically your melanocytes throwing their toys out of the pram. In a skin with melasma the melanocytes are going off like fireworks.

Best product choice: time, a package of laser treatments, supportive products for pigmentation, and sun block. I had mild melasma with pregnancy: it eventually cleared up on its own, but some people aren't that lucky. Clinical peels can help, but if you want it gone, you need the laser. And the bad news is that even if you stay out of the sun and wear a complete sunblock, it will probably come back, because that's what it does. It is also heat-triggered, so stay away from saunas and steam rooms.

Make sure you know whether you have melasma or pigmentation before you part with your hard-earned cash.

TRY THESE...

- Biologique Recherche P50 PIGM 400
- Murad Rapid Age Spot Correcting Serum
- NIOD RE:Pigment
- OSKIA Renaissance Brightlight Serum
- Renée Rouleau Advanced Resurfacing Serum
- Summer Fridays CC Me Serum
- The Ordinary Alpha Arbutin 2% + HA
- Zelens Lumino Brightening Serum

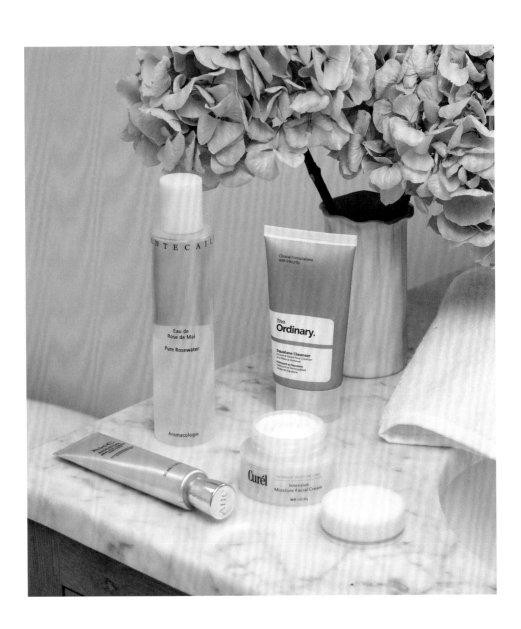

SKINCARE MYTH

EYE PRODUCTS FIX GENETIC DARK CIRCLES

Are dark circles driving you mad? Have you tried everything under the sun to get rid of them?

> Your options are limited in terms of what you can do about them, and there are definitely things that can make them worse.

I'm talking specifically to my lovely Asian readers, darker-skin-toned readers and even my red-headed, extremely pale readers. If you can see dark circles under your eyes and, to your knowledge, there is no particular reason for them, look at your parents/immediate family. If they also have dark circles, they probably run in your genes, and there isn't a cream alive that will safely deal with that kind of dark circle.

Sure, there are excellent eye products that can take the edge off, and some brightening ones that will 'lift' the appearance of them, but anyone who looks you in the eye and says, 'This cream will absolutely fix your dark circles,' is either misinformed or not being completely straight with you. It's a little easier for those of us with occasional dark circles caused by things like illness, dehydration or too much of a good (bad) thing, but genes are hard to mess with.

If you really hate the dark circles, you could talk to a dermatologist about trough filler: a non-surgical procedure, it involves injecting the area with hyaluronic acid filler, which sits just under the skin and essentially hides the dark circles. For most people, one treatment will last 12–18 months.

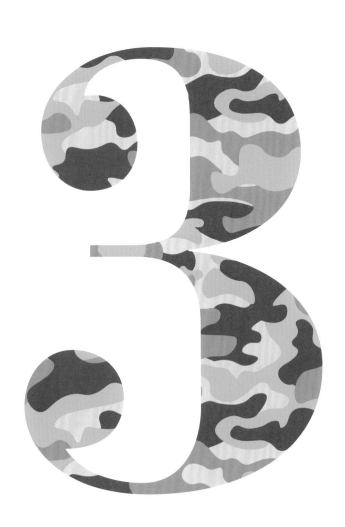

WHAT YOU NEED

"

THE FILLING OF THE SANDWICH IS MORE IMPORTANT THAN THE BREAD

"

WHAT YOU NEED

Now that you know what to do and when to do it, what do you use?

Your skincare kit deserves consideration and a bit of care. Like a bra or a haircut, it's personal to you and is going to see you through the next few months. Its effects are visible every single day, even if they are not obvious.

Skin health – and good skincare – is for life.

Your skin's not a designer handbag. You should be buying products for the formula and the ingredients, not the label, however much you like how the packaging looks. The previous pages should have given you a good idea of the issues you personally have to contend with, and the ingredients that you need to look out for. You should also have a better idea of how to tell if a product is working for you.

When choosing your products, whether you're just starting out in the world of skincare or are a seasoned pro, you need to shop in a way that's financially sustainable; that means not splurging on one 'luxury' product that you then save for 'best'. And on the flip side, you shouldn't be so busy looking to save pennies that you cut corners where you really should be investing. I'll say it again – invest in the middle of your routine where you can. And remember, keep everything (except your cleansing products) out of your bathroom – bathrooms are generally too hot.

This chapter is devoted to your kit. What each product does, where to invest and where you can save if you need to. Follow these rules and you'll soon find that not only are you making the most of every last bit of your product, but you might find you're actually enjoying yourself.

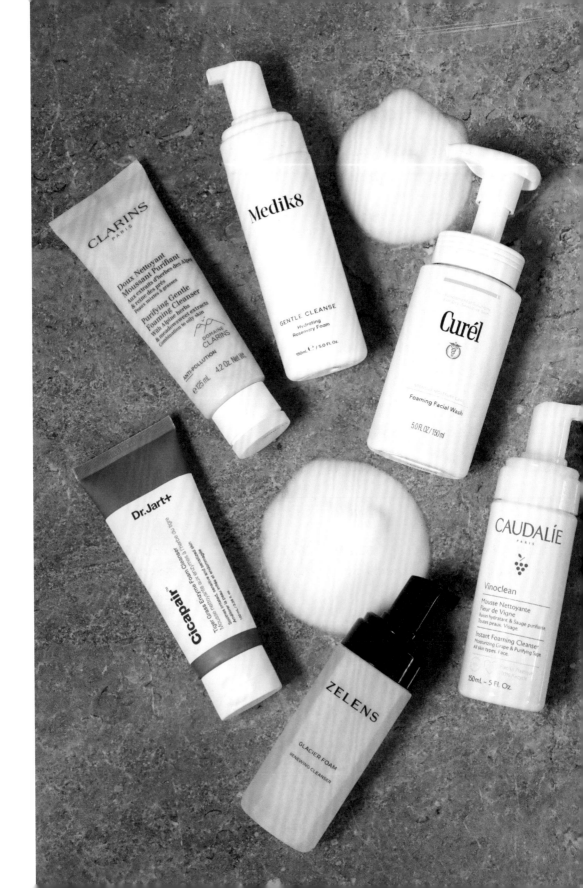

#1: CLEANSE

> Cleansing is **by far** the most important step of your routine.

If you are consistently 'cleansing' with wipes (aka moving the dirt around your face) and then applying a really expensive serum or moisturiser on top, you are wasting your money. And your time.

'Double cleansing' may be something that you are doing already in the evenings, this is just what I call it.

Essentially, if you are using more than one product to remove your makeup in the evenings, you are double cleansing.

For example, if you remove your eye makeup with a micellar water or eye-makeup remover before you cleanse, that is your first cleanse. You follow with a proper cleanser to remove everything else. That was your second cleanse.

NOTE: a micellar water is not your second cleanse. Stop that nonsense.

Let's be clear on something – there is no double cleansing in the mornings. Wake up, cleanse once, you're good to go. You have no makeup or SPF to remove. Crack on.

There is a trend for 60-second cleansing, meaning you apply all your cleanser, massage it around for 60 seconds, and remove. And you only do this once. That's fine if you want to do it in the mornings, but for the evening? I'm not a fan. If you are wearing makeup and SPF it is far less irritating to the skin to do two quicker cleanses than one long one. Loosen and remove the topical makeup/SPF with your first cleanse and clean your skin with the second one.

MORNING CLEANSE

Use any of the following:

- Gels
- Milks
- Lotions
- Balm cleansers
- Oils
- Clay-based cleansers

Basically, *anything* except:

- Wipes
- Micellar water

The morning cleanse routine is dependent on how your skin feels when you wake up and what you are doing with the rest of your day. For example, if I have a long day ahead of wearing makeup, I will probably use an oil to cleanse. My skin feels soft and holds moisture for longer afterwards, which has a knock-on effect on the rest of my routine and stops my makeup going patchy by the afternoon.

If I'm based at home for the day I'll use something slightly more 'active', follow with a strong acid toner and apply some treatment serums and heavier moisturisers.

If you know you are going to be based at home for the day and not wearing makeup, treat your skin as if it's a spa day: **cleanse, exfoliate, treat, repeat** (repeat the treat, not the entire routine!).

This is why my skin looks great if I've had a few consecutive days working from home, and looks merely 'okay' if I've had appointments in town every day of the week. And do not get me started on travelling... that's a whole other subject (see pages 174–175).

Wipes and micellar water are not suitable for mornings because you use them in an emergency or when removing makeup, and you won't be wearing makeup to bed, will you?

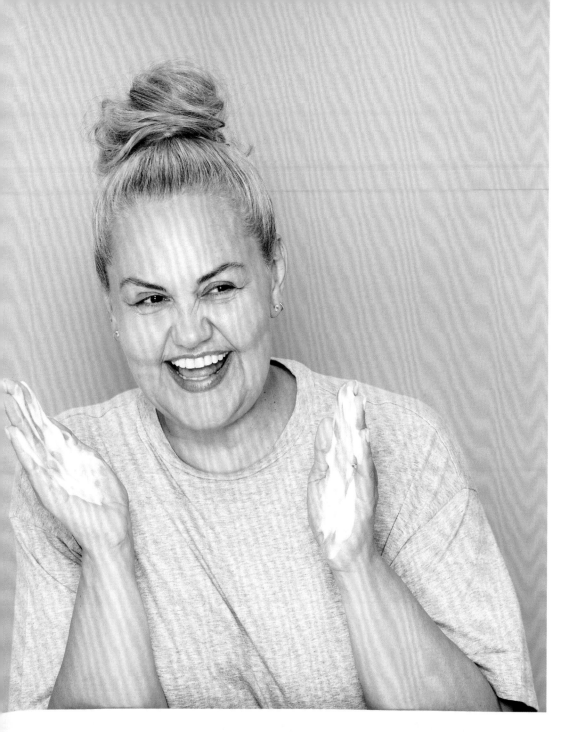

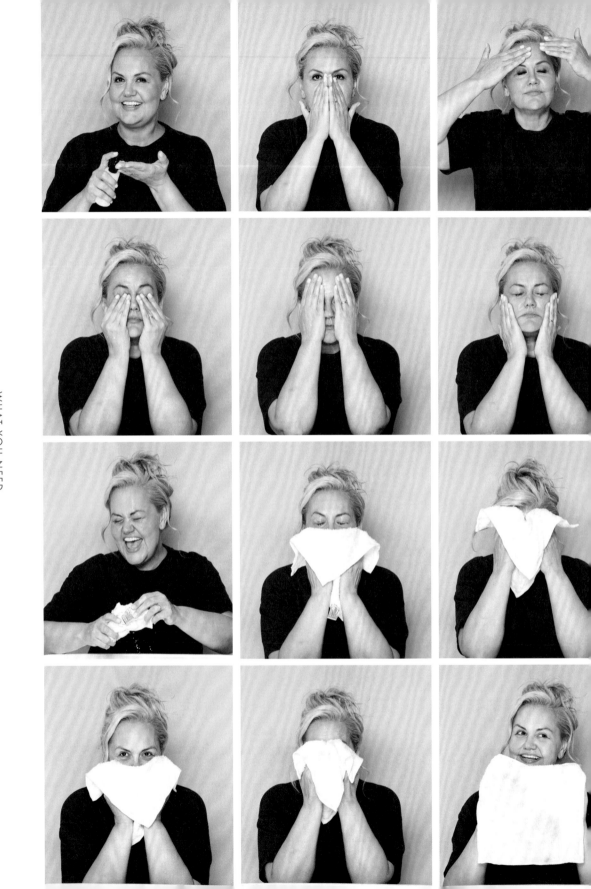

EVENING (DOUBLE) CLEANSE

Do what *you* need to do to remove what you've put on your face. You know your face/routine better than anyone on a beauty counter. Or me.

Wearing a ton of eye makeup? Remove it first.

Slathered in SPF? Take care of that first.

Both? Go in with grease. **When in doubt, go in with grease.** Think of all the old Hollywood movie stars and the footage of them removing their face with grease. It works. Just look at the last picture on the grid opposite – you know you're going to need to go in again with more cleanser and a rinsed-out cloth.

FIRST CLEANSE:

- Eye-makeup removers
- Micellar waters
- Greasy balms – not necessarily expensive ones, just ones that do a great job of removing makeup
- Cleansing creams – preferably thicker ones with a good oil content
- Oils – oils are great for removing makeup, but you don't have to pick a really expensive one for the first cleanse

SECOND CLEANSE:

This is where you use your most expensive cleansing product. This one is your skin cleanser more than your makeup remover. Its job is to make sure your skin is clean, balanced and comfortable and ready for everything else that you are applying afterwards. It's time to use your good stuff.

Some people are saying that double cleansing means using oil followed by foam. No.

You can obviously use one cleanser for both cleanses if you have budget concerns. We've all been there. Well, I certainly have. Just buy the best that you can afford, when you can afford it.

If you are using one product, apply a small amount for the first cleanse mainly to loosen eye makeup and product on cheek areas (where we tend to apply the most SPF). Remove with a flannel and go in again with another round.

The second cleanse is the massage stage, not the first. Don't spend a lot of time on your first cleanse. It's loosening the dirt, not vacuuming it all up.

The best products for second cleanse are:

- Cleansing balms: good ones. Gorgeous, plant-based, greasy ones. Greasy in the best way.
- Cleansing milks
- Cleansing gels (without SLS)
- Cleansing creams
- Cleansing clays
- Cleansing oils: oils and balms are easily my favourite choice for skin cleansing. They are brilliant for ensuring that everything is off and don't disturb the acid mantle (see Glossary) in an aggressive manner.

See page 118 for my recommendations of brands and products.

That is really all there is to it.

The important part is to remember to cleanse properly every single day without fail.

'PAT DRY'

This may seem like a strange one, so the context is important. I am always asked about routines and what order products should be used in.

There are some things that make it onto packaging purely because NPD (new product development) and marketing departments regurgitate the same advice time and time again, just because it's what they've done before.

One of the main culprits is on cleanser packaging, or in cleansing routines, when it says that after cleansing, you should 'rinse off, then pat dry'.

If you're soaking wet after a shower, you may want to lightly dry your face, mainly so you can see, but here's the thing: in an ideal world, you want a damp face.

If you use your flannels and follow my routines, your skin will be damp once you've cleansed. You need to go from there right to the next stage. Whether that's acids or spritzes. There's no need to pat dry first. Go straight in – a damp skin is a great skin to work on. Seal in the moisture with your following products.

There is one big exception: vitamin A.

Retinoids, especially prescription-strength ones, should be applied to dry skin after cleansing. I cleanse, use a flannel, then leave my skin to air-dry for a few minutes (usually just the time it takes to make tea; not hours) before I apply the retinoid, then I put other products on top (see pages 136–137).

KNOW YOUR CLEANSERS

A cleanser's job is to gently remove all the makeup, dirt and grime from your face. Cleansers are best chosen with your lifestyle in mind, while also paying attention to your skin concerns.

BALMS OR OILS

These are great for makeup and SPF removal – an oily/acne skin might find them too heavy or problematic to remove. I tend to use these for a first cleanse in the evening.

CREAMS

These do a great job of both removing makeup and cleansing the skin and are made for all skin types.

MILK OR LOTIONS

Traditionally used by French beauty houses, milks are runny, soft, easy to use and remove makeup and SPF and cleanse your skin.

GELS

Popular as a morning cleanse or a second cleanse in the evening (see page 40), gels are the preferred texture for a lot of people with combination/oily skin.

MICELLAR WATER

Micellar waters are a mixture of oil and water that are used as a liquid makeup remover. They should only be used as a first cleanse. Micellar waters are not ideal for regular use, or for cleaning the skin.

> In general, foaming is what you want washing-up liquid to do, not your cleanser. The old-school foaming products are NOT best for acne.

TRY THESE...

- Beauty Pie Japanfusion™ Pure Transforming Cleanser or Plantastic™ Apricot Butter Cleansing Balm

- Clinique Take The Day Off™ Cleansing Balm

- Deviant Cleansing Concentrate

- Emma Hardie Moringa Cleansing Balm

- Joanna Vargas Vitamin C Face Wash

- Jordan Samuel Skin The After Show Treatment Cleanser for Sensitive Skin

- OSKIA Renaissance Cleansing Gel

- Plenaire Rose Jelly Gentle Makeup Remover

- Tata Harper – all her cleansers!

- The Body Shop Camomile Sumptuous Cleansing Butter

- The Ordinary Squalane Cleanser

- Then I Met You Living Cleansing Balm

SPRITZES

Facial mists and sprays are an easy and affordable way to ensure that your skin stays hydrated without the need for heavier products. They are ideal as either a second tone (spritz) or just your general tone for those of you that don't use acids and/or on days you aren't using acids. Use them alone, after cleansing, under serums, over serums, under moisturiser, over moisturiser, under makeup, over makeup, on an airplane, in your car, at your desk, when it's hot, when it's cold... wherever and whenever. If in doubt, SPRITZ.

Some are water with added minerals such as zinc and magnesium, while others (which tend to be more expensive) have added peptides, rice bran oils, rose oils etc. – just more 'oomph'. Hyaluronic acid and glycerin can usually be found in them, along with other hydrating factors.

They are variously labelled as 'hydrating mists', 'spritzes', 'essences' and 'face sprays'.

TRY THESE...

- Curél Deep Moisture Spray
- Dr.Jart+™ Cicapair™ Tiger Grass Calming Mist
- January Labs Restorative Tonic Mist
- Josh Rosebrook Hydrating Accelerator
- La Roche-Posay Toleriane Ultra 8 Face Mist
- La Roche-Posay Serozinc
- Mother Dirt AO+ Mist
- VENeffect Skin Calming Mist

MICELLAR WATERS ARE A 'PROPER' CLEANSER

I am tagged on Twitter or Instagram on a daily basis whenever there is an article singing the praises about micellar waters, particular cleansers or wipes (God – always the wipes!), online or in a magazine. I read as many of them as I can: sometimes they make me laugh, sometimes I find I agree with them. But, articles describing micellar water as a cleanser never do.

Micellar waters were originally designed to be used for those occasional times when you have no access to water, like backstage at fashion shows (hence the huge awareness of Bioderma) or at a festival (see pages 168–172).

Firstly, I will never for the life of me understand why some people think that using these products is 'quicker' than washing your face. If using micellar water is 'quicker' than washing your face, you're using it incorrectly. A quick swipe across the forehead is not going to clean your face. When I have to use them backstage at shows it takes me at least four sets of two separate cotton pads to clean the face of makeup. Using both sides. That's not quick. Add to that the constant rubbing of cotton wool and ingredients that aren't exactly 'softening' and you're setting yourself up for a sore face.

These waters are ingredient-heavy, some contain alcohol and most contain fragrance. Before those of you that have to use micellar waters jump to their defence, as I've already said, do what you have to.

> Work situations, new babies, flying, the gym – micellar waters can come in handy. But try to make them a temporary substitute, not a permanent fixture.

121

#2: TREAT

Once your face is clean, you're free to start treating your current skin condition (see page 69). Depending on the needs of your skin, and your time constraints and chosen budget, this list of needs can be as long or as short as you want it to be.

ACIDS

I understand that combining the words 'acid' and 'skin' can potentially be intimidating. Don't be scared! Acids aren't actually that new. One of the first acid toners, P50 by Biologique Recherche, has been going since 1970. I've been banging on about them for ages, and thankfully they've gained in momentum in recent years.

Acids are all about exfoliation, and are derived from professional chemical peels, but are now included in our everyday skincare routines. I originally coined the phrase 'acid toning' to allow readers to easily identify where it goes in their routine i.e. after cleansing – the liquid acid stage basically replaces your traditional toner.

ACIDS OVERVIEW

LACTIC (AHA) – resurfacing, great for dehydrated and dry skin.

GLYCOLIC (AHA) – stimulating for better collagen production, resurfacing.

MALIC (AHA) – resurfacing, good for boosting collagen production.

SALICYLIC (BHA) – best for spots/acne. Surprisingly gentle.

POLYHYDROXY (PHA) – best for those in need of hydration and deep penetration of a product applied afterwards.

Try to buy two, preferably three, acid products: a strong one for evenings, a lighter one for daytime and one more to mix it up. Different strengths and different acids do different things to the skin, and you'll want to tweak which you use depending on how your skin's feeling.

All acids are available in a variety of strengths, and come in many forms: liquids, pre-soaked pads and gels.

There are three main types of acid:

ALPHA HYDROXY ACIDS (AHAs)

These are the most commonly used acids and include glycolic, citric, mandelic, malic, tartaric and lactic. They exfoliate the skin, stimulate collagen and GAGs (glycosaminoglycans) formation. They normalise the stratum corneum (the outer-most layer of the epidermis) and can regulate keratinisation. They are best for targeting signs of ageing.

You need these if *your skin is showing signs of ageing.*

BETA HYDROXY ACID (BHA)

There is only one beta hydroxy acid – salicylic. It is derived from acetylsalicylic acid, or willow bark. Like AHAs, beta hydroxy acid (BHA) also acts as an exfoliant, increasing the shedding of dead skin cells. BHA is extremely useful for treating breakouts and helps manage keratosis pilaris and other conditions that involve blocked or clogged pores.

You need this if *you suffer with blemishes, spots or acne.*

POLYHYDROXY ACIDS (PHAs)

The next generation of AHAs, these allow for slower and gradual penetration. The absorption is non-irritating and doesn't sting. PHAs support the matrix around collagen, help restore skin barrier function and protect against collagen degradation. PHAs are probably the most multi-tasking of all acids. Gluconolactone, lactobionic and maltobionic are examples of PHAs. They are best for targeting signs of ageing, and using on sensitive or dehydrated skins.

You need these if *your skin is sensitive but you want the effects of acid.*

But that's not the end of it. Within these categories, acids can be broken down into even more types, depending on what they're made from.

GLYCOLIC ACID (AHA)

Containing the smallest molecule in AHAs, glycolic acid is derived from sugarcane and is the most effective AHA due to its ability to penetrate deeply and stimulate fibroblast cells (see Glossary) to aid in collagen production. It exfoliates the skin by increasing cell turnover, helps even out skin tone and builds the support structure in the dermal matrix, which in turn reduces the appearance of wrinkles. It is the only acid that makes you more sun-sensitive.

You need this if *you are over 30 or 35 and your main concern is ageing.*

LACTIC ACID (AHA)

Historically derived from milk, lactic acid has more recently been synthetically formed to maintain its stability in products. Lactic acid works to dissolve the glue in between cells on the surface, making it good for gently exfoliating. It keeps the skin soft and acts like Pac Man on the surface of the skin, gently eating it away.

You need this if *your main concern is dull, dehydrated or dry skin.*

WHAT'S THE MAIN DIFFERENCE BETWEEN THEM?

AHAs are water-soluble and, with the exception of glycolic acid, they do not penetrate deeply beneath the skin's surface.

BHA is oil- (lipid-) soluble. This allows the BHA to penetrate oily pores and help to exfoliate the pore itself. This is why salicylic is particularly useful for oily and acneic skins.

PHAs tend to be better for sensitive skins due to their larger molecular size and slower penetration. PHAs are great humectants (they attract moisture to the skin), making them particularly good choices for dehydrated skins.

"

USING ACID TONERS IS LIKE TAKING YOUR FACE TO THE GYM

"

MANDELIC ACID (AHA)

Fat-soluble and derived from almonds, this is a good choice for oilier skins, as the molecules can penetrate even the greasiest skin. Mandelic acid is antibacterial and, with regular usage, can reduce oiliness without harshly drying out the skin.

You need this if *your skin is on the oilier side, but you don't particularly suffer with spots (can happily be used with a BHA).*

CITRIC ACID (AHA)

May help to reverse the signs of photo/sun damage, while also improving the quality of the dermal matrix. It's mostly used at preservative level, just so brands can list it on the ingredients label. Look for specific mentions of citric acid in the descriptions on packaging: if they're not there, it's probably used as a preservative only. You don't need to seek out citric acid especially, but it is used in a lot of formulas.

TARTARIC AND MALIC ACID (AHAs)

Mainly derived from grapes, apples, pears and cherries, these two are gentler on the AHA scale but do act as antioxidants and aid skin respiration. You wouldn't seek these out in particular, as they're not key ingredients.

SALICYLIC ACID (BHA)

Derived from willow bark, salicylic acid is oil-soluble and penetrates and breaks down the 'glue' that causes breakouts and oily, uneven skins. It loosens desmosomes, allowing the cell to let go of the excess sebum that oily skins like to hold on to (think of desmosomes as handcuffs, attaching your cells together – salicylic acid unlocks the handcuffs).

You need this if *you suffer from spots. If you live in Europe, this is your alternative to benzoyl peroxide.*

GLUCONOLACTONE ACID (PHA)

A largely antioxidant PHA, gluconolactone is the multi-tasker of all acids. It is made of multiple humectant hydroxyls, which hydrate the skin. It also attacks free radicals, protecting the skin from UV damage and strengthening barrier function, allowing the skin to reduce in redness with regular use. Gluconolactone inhibits elastase, the cause of skin sagging, and helps maintain elasticity.

You need this if *you have sensitive skin. It plays well with others.*

LACTOBIONIC ACIDS (PHAs)

Derived from milk sugars, lactobionic acids are antioxidants. They help prevent and reverse signs of ageing including lines, pigmentation, large pores and uneven skin texture, promote skin firmness and stop the degradation of collagen. A natural humectant, they bind water to the skin.

You need these if *you're dehydrated.*

MALTOBIONIC ACID (PHA)

The most humectant of acids, maltobionic acid gives antioxidant protection, protects skin from hyperpigmentation caused by sun exposure, and helps prevent collagen degradation. Maltobionic acid can improve skin texture, firmness, clarity and tone, and reduce the appearance of wrinkles. You'll see it in an ingredients list, but don't need to seek it out particularly. It's good if your skin is dry or dehydrated.

THE OTHER 'ACIDS'

Azelaic and hyaluronic acids, although 'acids', are not exfoliating, and so are not in this section. They're just not that kind of acid.

TRY THESE...

- Biologique Recherche Lotion P50 (various)
- Deviant Gentle Resurfacing Liquid
- Dr. Dennis Gross Alpha Beta® Peel (various strengths available)
- First Aid Beauty Facial Radiance Pads

- OSKIA Liquid Mask
- Josh Rosebrook Daily Acid Toner
- Kate Somerville Liquid ExfoliKate®
- Pestle & Mortar NMF Lactic Acid Toner

ACID MYTHS

Some of the most frequent questions I am asked concern acids, specifically glycolic acid. So, let's clear a few things up:

MYTH: Glycolic thins the skin.
FACT: Glycolic acid thickens the skin. Glycolic acid exfoliates and thins the outer stratum corneum (the pleasingly named 'horny layer') of your skin, making it more flexible. It also restores the essential components of the skin that are damaged as we age, leading to an increase in collagen fibre density (and therefore thicker skin) that then functions more youthfully. For smoother-textured, softer, younger-looking skin, more evenness of skin tone and clarity, and a fuller, firmer skin with more elasticity and less laxity, use glycolic acid.

MYTH: You must use SPF30 or above if using acids, as AHAs increase sensitivity to UV light.
FACT: Increases in sunburn cell formation have been documented following AHA use, however this effect can be prevented by use of the very lowest level of sunscreen, even as low as an SPF2.

* This fact is merely to reassure you that if you use acids, you're not burning your face off when you go outside. It's not to encourage you to cease SPF usage, which you will still need for the usual reasons.*

MYTH: AHAs diminish skin barrier function.
FACT: US FDA studies have not shown an increase in the absorption of studied materials, which means that skin barrier function is not decreased. Further studies have demonstrated AHA-related improvements in skin barrier function.

MYTH: AHAs cause skin irritation.
FACT: AHAs are known to occasionally produce transient stinging, especially at higher strengths. The stinging should be fleeting and should not produce excessive redness. Mild irritation can be (but is not always) part of the process.

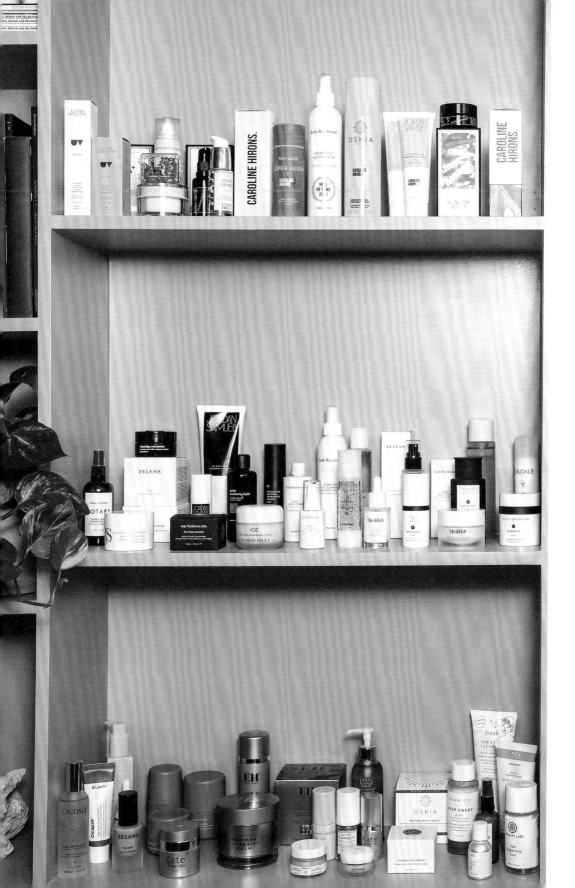

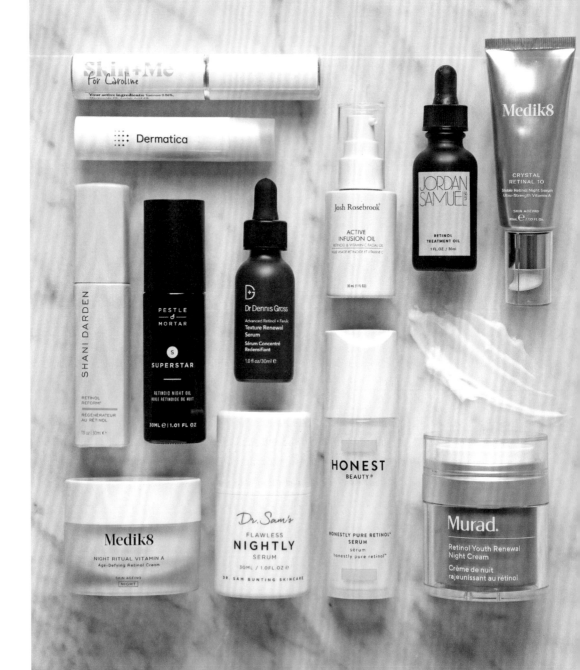

VITAMIN A AND RETINOID PRODUCTS

This is one of the products I'm most frequently asked about, and potentially one of the most confusing. All you need to know is that it's ALL VITAMIN A. In the same way that white sugar, brown sugar and maple syrup are all sugar, retinoid is the family name for any vitamin A product. Other ways you might see this ingredient listed on packaging are: retinol, retinal, retinyl palmitate, tretinoin, retinaldehyde, retinyl retinoate, hydroxypinacolone retinoate or adapalene.

> Originally discovered as having beneficial side effects when treating acne, vitamin A is widely considered to be the gold standard of skincare because it is scientifically proven not only to reverse the signs of ageing, but also shown to prevent them.

A lot of people contact me because they're scared to try a vitamin A product, or they used it once, had a bad reaction and are worried about going back to it. There are side effects to using vitamin A products, but with correct usage, there is nothing on the market that gives the same results on the skin.

HOW TO USE

- Use after cleansing, and make sure your skin is dry before you start.

- General guidance is to use vitamin A in the evening, but some newer formulas state that they can be used during the day.

- Always use an SPF (in your morning routine).

- Start with a milder percentage and work your way up. The percentage will vary depending on the type of retinoid (see pages 134–135).

- Generally one full cycle (one tube or jar) of a product is enough to build up resistance and move up to the next strength.

- Less is more. You will be directed to use a pea-sized amount of prescription-strength formulas, however you can use a little more of OTC formulas.

- Avoid the eyes, the area around the nostrils, corners of the mouth and be gentle with the neck (see page 137).

Most people are put off using a vitamin A product because they weren't told how their skin would initially react. Vitamin A, at its core, is designed to resurface the skin, stimulate collagen production and reverse the signs of ageing. This doesn't happen overnight, and might require a bit of a journey. It can be a shock if you were expecting to wake up 10 years younger, but actually you might wake up looking like you've had an allergic reaction, but it is worth it – it just takes a little while to get there.

WHAT TO EXPECT WHEN YOU START

- Redness
- Dryness
- Patches of flaking skin
- Generally irritated skin (in varying degrees, depending on the formula)

I'm really selling it to you, aren't I? This reaction is completely normal and to be expected. To encourage you to keep going, this is what you do while your skin is acclimatising.

- Your first port of call is to buffer the product. This means weakening the formula by adding in a layer of moisturiser either before or after you apply the retinol.

- Avoid foaming products, especially cleansers, as they will be too drying.

- Avoid powders and heavy foundations. They will make the flaking look SO much worse. I refer to my skin as 'sausage roll pastry' when it's at this stage. However, life goes on and if you want to wear makeup, you need a really good moisturiser instead of a primer. I've found Embryolisse Lait-Crème Concentré works really well for me. The mineral oil base, on this occasion, is a plus, as it stops your skin from taking the water from your foundation and going flaky and patchy.

- Oils are your friend. Squalane and jojoba oils are really light and, unlike some heavier oils, won't stop the retinol from working. When I'm using retinols, I have a squalane oil on me at all times and use it throughout the day.

WHAT TO EXPECT ONCE YOUR SKIN ACCLIMATISES

- Smoother skin
- Glowing skin
- Fewer visible lines
- Better skin tone and elasticity
- Plumper skin
- More hydrated skin

HOW OFTEN SHOULD YOU USE IT?

As the great Kate Somerville says, use your vitamin A according to the decade you're in. If you're in your 20s, use it twice a week; 30s, three times a week; 40s, four times a week; and so on.

WHEN WILL YOU SEE THE EFFECTS?

In line with your age, and how much there is to repair, how quickly you'll see results will vary.

- Over 40: 1 month
- 30–40: 2 weeks
- 20–30: strangely longer, as you don't have much to fix

Because the side effects do not show on your skin immediately, you may be tempted to use more than suggested, and apply it more frequently. Do not do this. Seriously. I mean it.

Don't.

HOW DO YOU KNOW IF YOU'VE OVERDONE IT?

- Somebody says, 'Oh my god, what has actually happened to your face?'

- Your normal moisturiser stings.

- Your skin feels burned and is sore. This is beyond dry or uncomfortable. It is literally painful to the touch. A gust of wind would make you wince and you feel like your face is going to fall off.

- It's sore around your nostrils or the corners of your eyes and eyelids.

- Blistering/bleeding (just stop already).

The severity of your reaction, and how long you attempted to use vitamin A for before stopping, will dictate how soon you can try again. Apply a lot of nourishing products while your skin recovers, give it a couple of weeks or longer for your skin to return to normal, then try it again once more, but buffer it and go slowly.

A ROUGH GUIDE TO RETINOIDS

There are plenty of vitamin A derivatives in formulas but these are the main characters you should be inviting to the party:

THE BOSS

Tretinoin (retinoic acid/all trans-retinoic acid), aka 'Tret', is available as prescription-strength products only. It comes in three strengths and you will work up from 0.025% to 0.05% and finally 0.1%, guided by your dermatologist. It is suitable for most skin types.
POTENTIAL FOR IRRITATION: high

THE HEAVYWEIGHT

Not the boss but it packs a punch, **retinaldehyde** is the next level down from retinoic acid. It acts quickly on the skin, but can be irritating. It is clinically proven to work up to 11 times faster than retinol. Suitable for older skins that want quick results.
POTENTIAL FOR IRRITATION: medium

THE NEW KID ON THE BLOCK

Retinyl retinoate (RR), less well known than HPR, is the child of retinoic acid and retinol. It's a fairly new addition to the family, and has been shown to be more stable and more active than retinol, causing less irritation. Suitable for sensitive skins.
POTENTIAL FOR IRRITATION: low to medium

THE COUSIN

Related to The Boss but not a direct descendant, **hydroxypinacolone retinoate** (HPR) is more of a cousin to its stronger relative. It is sometimes offered in higher percentages because it's an ester (i.e. it's oil-based), and therefore more gentle. Suitable for sensitive skins.
POTENTIAL FOR IRRITATION: low

THE TEENAGER

I call **retinol** the teenager because it's often irritating, in varying strengths. Having said that, retinol is the most widely available vitamin A in over-the-counter products. It is generally available in 0.3%, 0.5% and 1%. It works in the same way as the stronger ingredients above – it just takes you longer to get there. Suitable for all skin types.
POTENTIAL FOR IRRITATION: high, depending on the percentage

THE LINEKER (YEAH, I'M A FOOTBALL FAN)

Adapalene (trade name Differin) plays well with others and has never been sent off, and is available over the counter in the USA. It is mainly used for acne but has proven benefits on signs of ageing on the skin, so is a good pick if you are Stateside and looking for something easy to access that won't break the bank or your skin. Suitable for all skin types, but especially useful for acne or breakouts.
POTENTIAL FOR IRRITATION: fairly low

TRY THESE VITAMIN A BRANDS

- Beauty Pie
- Medik8
- Murad
- Paula's Choice
- SkinCeuticals

HOW TO USE A VITAMIN A PRODUCT

Brands will all provide you with individual instructions on the packaging. While there will always be exceptions, the key things to remember are:

- **Do not apply a lot, thinking it will work faster.** It won't. Save your money, and your skin. Apply a small, pea-sized amount, or in the case of an oil, a few drops, not an entire pipette. The results can be very alarming (in a good way – you may notice the difference almost overnight). Do not be tempted to think more is more. It isn't. In the case of vitamin A, and especially if you have not used a vitamin A product before, less is more.

- **Use it every third night,** moving to more regular use when you know your skin is tolerating it (unless a brand specifically says differently). This analogy might be helpful: if you're in your 30s, try to use it 3 times a week; if you're in your 40s, go for 4 times a week; and in your 50s, aim for daily use.

- **If in doubt,** apply your retinoid after cleansing, leave it on for 20–30 minutes by itself, then follow with either a soothing moisturiser or facial oil.

I have been using vitamin A products for a long time. If I know I'm using an OTC (over-the-counter) vitamin A product in the evening, I cleanse, sometimes acid tone (although less so if I am using a high-percentage retinoid), spritz, then apply my retinoid. If, however, I'm using a prescription-strength retinoid, I cleanse and then apply the cream.

I love retinoid products. They are easily the best products for fighting signs of ageing. Everyone should use one. They are worth the faff. Just use them correctly.

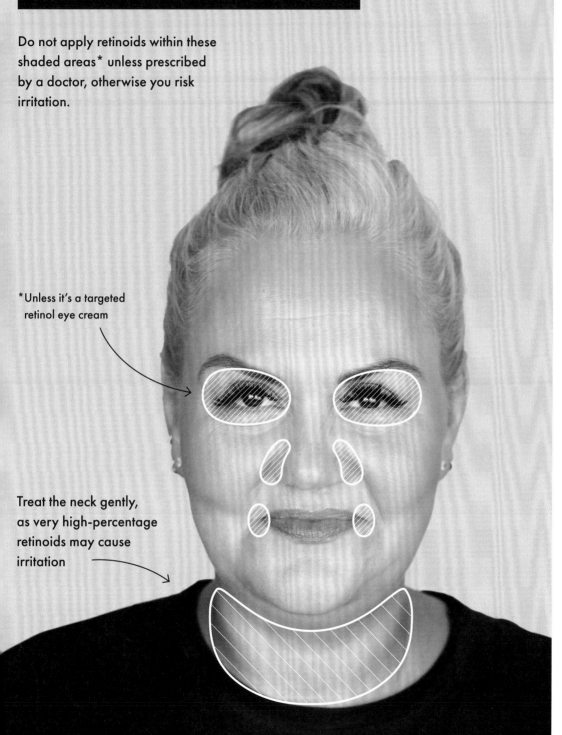

WHERE *NOT* TO PUT IT

Do not apply retinoids within these shaded areas* unless prescribed by a doctor, otherwise you risk irritation.

*Unless it's a targeted retinol eye cream

Treat the neck gently, as very high-percentage retinoids may cause irritation

EYE PRODUCTS

There are two camps when it comes to eye products: those who enjoy using them and see the benefits, and those who think they're unnecessary and a waste of money.

I am very much in the former camp. An eye cream or serum has been part of my routine since my 20s. I didn't start earlier because I was pretty healthy – I never smoked, didn't drink much alcohol – but once I was pregnant with my first child (at 22) I changed my mind.

The saying 'the eyes are the window to the soul' is derived from similar medical terms meaning the eyes are *literally* the window to what is going on inside the body. If you are blessed with youth and spectacular health your eyes are, I'm sure, clear and bright, and the skin around the orbicularis oculi area (think panda eye) evenly toned and coloured. However, for *most* of us the above is no longer the case. **Everything** affects your eye area and the health of all of your internal organs is reflected in them…

- **Liver problems:** yellow eyes
- **Problems with your lymph drainage system:** puffy, dark circles
- **General mild illness:** dull eyes
- **On medication** (especially antibiotics): discoloured, puffy, dull, dehydrated
- **Smoking:** grey, dehydrated
- **Lack of sleep/too much sleep:** puffy, dark circles, grey 'tired' eyes
- **Too much salt, caffeine and alcohol:** puffy, dark circles, dehydrated
- **Sun damage/ageing:** wrinkles, dehydrated

It's a minefield. The bad news is that *any* topical cream would be hard pushed to magically fix the above. What it *will* do, however, especially when used with a concealer, is temporarily mask some of the above. Eye products often contain ingredients such as caffeine, green tea and peptides to target puffiness, dark circles and wrinkles. While we're on the subject – any ethical brand will advise you that the effect of a product will wear off if you discontinue use. **No eye product is a permanent 'fix'.**

I like a separate eye product for a number of reasons but mainly because I am extremely prone to puffy eyelids and dark circles. Both are genetic, and there's nothing I can do to fix them permanently (excluding surgery for the lids), but some things make them much worse, and the heavier formulations of most moisturisers are one of them. For that reason I like thin serums and dedicated formulations for eyes. If you are young, or have budget concerns, you can skip eye products and take your hydrating serums up to the orbital bone.

A FEW DOS AND DON'TS

- Do not use mineral oil around your eye area. It tends to make the area puffy, which is the opposite of what you want. Use only the lightest of serums on the eyelids, for the same reason.
- Do not be tempted to use more than the advised amount of cream – it's unnecessary, it could cause irritation and is a waste of money.
- If you have eczema or psoriasis in the eye area (which is very common) you can use thicker creams on the lids as you'll need them – depending on the severity of your condition, they may be prescribed by your doctor. Although you might find a nice organic balm somewhere, no skincare brand can legally claim to treat those medical conditions.
- Keep it simple – too much fragrance in a product can really irritate the eye area – your eye product does not need to smell nice.
- Most allergies to eye products and eyeshadows/mineral makeup are caused by an ingredient called **bismuth oxychloride**. It is used to give the shimmer/light-reflective 'glow' and is a big allergen. If you've never been able to use a particular eye cream *or* eyeshadow and had it blamed on 'your eyes' by a brand, check their INCI list: you'll probably see bismuth oxychloride on there. If your mineral makeup makes you itch, check the label.

TRY THESE...

- AHC Essential Real Eye Cream for Face
- Biossance Squalane + Peptide Eye Gel
- Glossier Bubblewrap Eye & Lip Plumping Cream
- Kate Somerville Line Release® Under Eye Repair Cream
- OSKIA Eye Wonder Serum

- Paula's Choice Clinical Ceramide-Enriched Firming Eye Cream
- Pestle & Mortar Recover Eye Cream
- StriVectin Intensive Eye Concentrate for Wrinkles PLUS
- Sunday Riley Auto Correct Brightening and Depuffing Eye Contour Cream

SERUMS

Serums are one of the most misunderstood and confused elements of the routine. So let's get down to basics. A serum is a product designed to deliver a high concentration of active ingredients directly into your skin. They are the last thing you apply before your moisturiser. And if you're going to spend money anywhere in your routine, it's best spent here.

Think of the serum as the 'treat'ment stage of your routine. The active ingredient you want will depend on the condition that you want to treat. So when buying products, check the label to see if the formula contains the suggested key ingredients for your skin type and condition (see Chapter 2).

Serums can be offered as oils, gels or lotions but are generally water-based. As a rule of thumb, apply the thinnest serums first, however there will always be exceptions, and reading labels is key.

TRY THESE...

These brands all make excellent serums for all skin concerns:

- Beauty Pie
- Kate Somerville
- La Roche-Posay
- Medik8
- Murad
- NIOD
- OSKIA
- SkinCeuticals
- The Ordinary
- Vichy
- Zelens

#3: MOISTURISE

This is the final hydrating step in your routine, before you apply SPF, and it's also the product that you don't need to blow your budget on. Moisturisers are generally classed in three categories:

EMOLLIENTS

These add oil to the epidermis and soften and smooth the skin, and are found in products aimed at dry skin.

HUMECTANTS

These attract water from the atmosphere and the epidermis and are found in most moisturisers. They are particularly beneficial for dehydrated and oilier skins.

OCCLUSIVES

These coat the stratum corneum (the outermost layer of the epidermis) and prevent transepidermal water loss (TEWL). They are generally recommended in a professional capacity for people suffering with skin conditions such as eczema or psoriasis.

TRY THESE...

- Avène Tolèrance Extrême Range
- Glossier Priming Moisturiser
- Jordan Samuel Skin The Performance Cream
- Josh Rosebrook Vital Balm Cream
- Kate Somerville Peptide K8® Power Cream
- May Lindstrom The Blue Cocoon
- Murad Hydro-Dynamic Ultimate Moisture
- OSKIA Bedtime Beauty Boost
- Pestle & Mortar Hydrate Lightweight Moisturiser
- REN Vita Mineral™ Daily Supplement Moisturising Cream

STEP AWAY FROM THE GLITTER

Glitter in skincare is just a downright nonsense. I don't know who started it. I don't care. It needs to end. And end now.

Glitter is a pain in the arse. It can be nice in an eyeshadow, when applied well. If you're a teen, knock yourself out: now is the time to swim in glitter if you want to. If you're in your 20s and enjoy a glittery face, again, knock yourself out. It's a legal requirement at festivals. I get it.

If, however, you are the rest of us, STOP. JUST MAKE IT STOP.

I mean, I don't know how much any of this needs saying, but there is ABSOLUTELY ZERO BENEFIT TO PUTTING GLITTER IN SKINCARE. If you have less-than-perfect skin, please stay away. It's also bad for the environment and will potentially lead to the next microbead situation (we can only hope brands will be responsible and remove it from their products before that happens).

If you want to take a fun selfie for social media wearing a glitter mask, that's your call. But DON'T. OKAY? DON'T. JUST DO NOT. I know some of you think it's fun, but the skincare community feels faint with despair at every new launch. And if you are a 'skincare' brand making money selling frigging glitter? Go sit in a dark room and think long and hard about your actions.

MOISTURISER IS YOUR MOST IMPORTANT PURCHASE

I've lost count of the number of times I've had a conversation with people who tell me they are using an incredibly expensive moisturiser, but cleansing (or not) with wipes or a quick wash in the shower.

Your moisturiser is your coat. It's your protection and 'cushion' from the elements.

Of course it's important – and yes, you can find moisturisers that contain all sorts of lovely wonderful things such as peptides, vitamins and other active ingredients, but those ingredients will generally work better for you in a serum where they can more freely penetrate and get to work while your moisturiser stands guard.

There is absolutely no point in buying the latest 'wonder' cream if you've done no prep work. If you spend a fair amount of cash on your cleansing routine, including acid toners, and a bit more on a serum, you can get away with saving your pennies on a moisturiser.

There are, of course, as with anything in life, exceptions. If you are 40+ it is potentially worthwhile using a high-tech moisturiser alongside your serum; one that also contains the 'active' ingredients found in your serum. Attack it from all angles by all means. If you are on a tight budget, prioritise your spending on exfoliating acids and a good retinoid serum and you can get away with cheaper cleansers and moisturisers.

How much time do you spend choosing your coat in the morning compared to picking your outfit?

Your cleanse-acid-serum routine is your 'outfit'. Put the work in and you'll see the results. Just don't forget your coat.

143

SHEET MASKS

'Sheet masks are wipes with holes
cut out for the eyes.'

When I tweeted this in 2018, it caused the skincare equivalent of Armageddon.

Some context: I'm not a massive fan of sheet masks, those single-use face-shaped pieces of polyfabric soaked in goodness-knows-what, that promise to saturate your skin with beneficial ingredients. Yes, I've used them, we all have. I've had the Instagram moment with my mum, daughter and I all doing them for the camera, but now I can't be bothered. They're wet, sticky and do not give you anything you can't get from applying a couple of rounds of hyaluronic acid serum to your face before your moisturiser.

At the risk of completely alienating everyone, I find I am hardly using any masks at all these days. I've got my skincare routine pretty nailed. If you find you need masks regularly, for anything other than pampering and comfort (not to be underestimated by any stretch), look at what needs tweaking in your daily routine as opposed to buying another product that you can only use sporadically in an attempt to fix it.

Now, obviously there are few notable exceptions – times when a mask makes sense:

Travel: I will occasionally use masks when travelling, especially flying (see pages 174–175), but in all honesty I get a better result from a hyaluronic acid serum and a good cream, with a hyaluronic acid mist used sporadically through the journey.

'Glow': I'm all for the occasional resurfacing boost, whether from a gentle exfoliating mask or an acidic mask. Everyone has dull days. But, if you find yourself reaching for them more frequently, you need to check your routine.

Spots: There is nothing more satisfying than putting a clay mask on spots. My teen daughter and her friends are obsessed with masking. They walk around the house with their clay-laden T-zones like they're wearing a badge of honour. As they should be at 18. But I haven't had that kind of skin in a long time. I don't get hormonal spots anymore. It's one of the joys of being closer to menopause than the age I started my periods. If I do get a whacking big, red angry spot, I'm far more likely to douse it in acid and oil until it gives in and goes away (see pages 232–235).

Honestly? That's about it. Maybe it's because I'm older. I'm definitely busier, and... I'm pathologically immune to trends.

Sheet masks aren't going anywhere, and sales of them are booming (considering their effects on the environment, this is not a good thing).

I'm merely suggesting that skincare, especially serums, has evolved to such a degree that you may not need masks. They're at the bottom of my 'kit' list. And if you do use them, bin them. They don't flush.

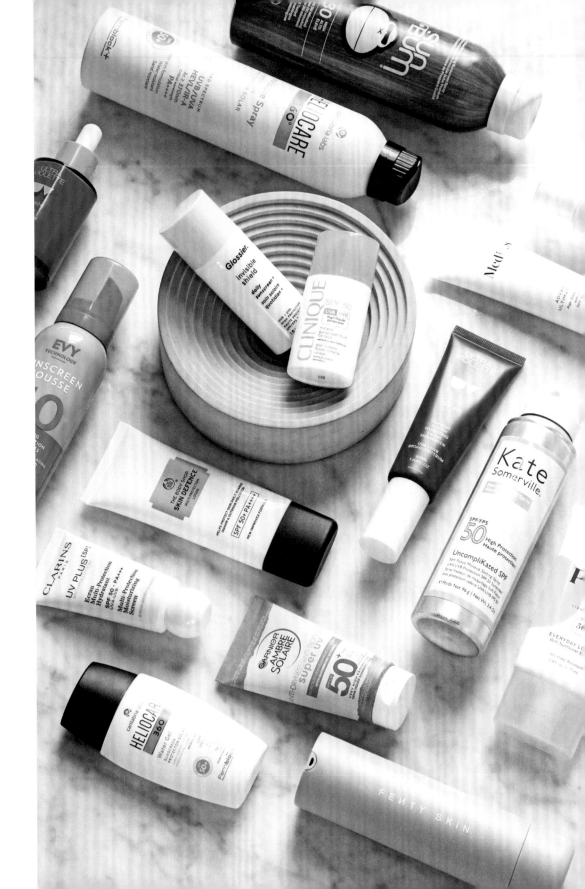

#4: PROTECT

Long gone are the days of my 80s youth, when I'd baste myself with baby oil on a foil suntanning sheet. These days, I wear an SPF50+ every day, and I haven't actually sat out in the sun for years.

SPF seems to always be in the news these days, so let's start with some SPF myth-busting. Almost as if we're burning sage and cleansing the area for fresh eyes.

'PHYSICAL' VS 'CHEMICAL'

SPF stands for Sun Protection Factor. If you have read anything about SPF in recent years you may have been told there are two types of sunscreen: **physical** and **chemical**.

A '**physical** sunscreen' is allegedly 'natural' and contained either zinc oxide or titanium dioxide as the UV filter.

A '**chemical** sunscreen' has been rather demonised in the press, but is basically the term used for a sunscreen that contains any other type of UV filter.

Physical sunscreens (ironically called 'inorganic' in scientific classification) are not, contrary to popular belief, 'natural'. Zinc oxide and titanium dioxide, which are most commonly used in 'natural' sunscreens, are not biodegradable and invariably use nanotechnology, which is being investigated by cancer research bodies because of its possible links to cancers in humans. If your preference is to use a 'natural' SPF, your closest bet is a 'non-nano' oxide. The term non-nano means nothing to the FDA, but it may be better for you. Bear in mind this is still technically a chemical, no matter what the 'green and clean' brigade say.

Chemical sunscreen (known as 'organic' in scientific classification) refers to any SPF on the market containing anything other than solely zinc oxide or titanium dioxide. They also absorb UV rays and produce heat by breaking them down in the skin. They have better, more modern filters and they're much nicer to use for people with darker skin tones as they don't leave a white cast.

HOW DOES SPF ACTUALLY WORK?

Traditionally, we have been told that 'chemical' SPFs absorb the light, while physical SPFs reflect it. We now know this not to be the case. They actually work in much the same way.

Just like 'chemical' sunscreens, mineral sunscreens work by absorbing the UV rays and turning them into heat. Around 90–95 per cent of the UV is absorbed by a mineral sunscreen, leaving only 5–10 per cent that is reflected/scattered. And when it is scattered, it just goes further into the skin, which is not a problem as the odds are it hits another patch of SPF and is absorbed. This however does make a mockery of all the visual aids you will frequently see from brands that show their mineral SPF deflecting the sun's rays like Wonder Woman with a shield. That's just not how this works.

There are two main concerns from being in the sun: skin-ageing and skin cancer.

UV light causes sunburn and sun damage by damaging cellular DNA.
UVA (long-wave) rays penetrate deep into the skin, gradually destroying elasticity and causing premature ageing. These rays penetrate glass.
UVB (short-wave) rays cause the burning and skin damage. They can alter the structure of skin cells, and ultimately lead to possible skin cancer.

Think A for ageing, B for burning

Both the US Department of Health and Human Services and the World Health Organization have identified UV light as a proven human carcinogen.

There is no such thing as a 'safe tan'.

A tan is a sign of DNA damage. It is the result of a chemical reaction in your body as it tries (and fails) to protect itself from UV light. Brands selling SPF that use the term 'safe tanning' are at best misleading, and at worst, clueless.

The majority of sun damage is done in the first 20 years of your life. Age spots and pigmentation that appear when you're older are the fault of those teen family holidays, not the tan you got last year.

"

THE MAJORITY OF SUN DAMAGE IS DONE IN YOUR FIRST 20 YEARS

"

HOW TO USE SPF

▎ Use a dedicated SPF.

In the past, I would get my SPF from my make-up, but since I've got older, and seen visible signs of ageing on my skin in the form of pigmentation and melasma, as well as using more actives, I've stepped up my SPF usage considerably. I use SPF50 daily: a dedicated sunscreen that gives both UVA and UVB protection. UVC doesn't penetrate the atmosphere, so we don't need to worry on that score.

I always recommend using a separate SPF. Although a moisturiser with added SPF obviously has to pass the same testing as a dedicated SPF, there are numerous problems with relying on a moisturiser with added SPF as your sun protection. Namely: you are less likely to apply it to all areas, you are more likely to apply only where you need moisturiser, and you are less likely to reapply a moisturiser during the day. What if you don't 'need' more moisturiser, but need to top up your SPF? For me, they fall under the category of a fallback, not something for daily use.

My problem with SPF in moisturisers is two-fold:

#1 **It gives you a false sense of security.** In the 1920s, when SPF wasn't available, the incidences of melanoma were around 1 in 1,500. In 2013, with years of SPF being available and modern science, the incidences are 1 in 53 – **1 in 53**. Why? Because we apply it once and move on, thinking we're done.

For example, let's say you use a moisturiser containing SPF15 at 8am, and would normally burn after 15 minutes of sun exposure. Technically you should be reapplying your SPF at 11.45am. And that's assuming you applied it all over your face – most people leave out areas when moisturising. How are you going to do that without removing your full face of makeup? I know no-one who takes their makeup off halfway through the day to reapply sunscreen.

And if you are sunbathing, to use the recommended amount of sunscreen you would need to use a bottle of that SPF15 moisturiser a day. A DAY.

If you apply your SPF moisturiser religiously every day and think you are protected, you may not be.

#2

A moisturiser containing SPF invariably only protects from UVB – it does not protect you from UVA. So, you won't burn, but your collagen will break down and you'll still get wrinkles. Excellent. Also – SPF moisturisers are less likely to be rub-resistant or water-resistant. If you then apply your makeup with fingers or a brush (everyone) or sweat, it's gone.

Companies that add SPF to their general 'anti-ageing' moisturisers are throwing it in there as an 'added benefit' and a sales tool.

Sun protection is not an 'added benefit'. It's a critical, proven step to protect from ageing.

Do not use an SPF instead of a moisturiser. That's like going out all day with a raincoat on and only bra and knickers underneath. Unless that is your everyday outfit of choice, I suggest you wear actual clothes (moisturiser) underneath your raincoat (SPF). There are obviously some caveats: newer SPFs contain great moisturising properties, and for some oilier or combination-skinned people, using an SPF without a moisturiser underneath may be enough for your skin.

Do not waste your money on a really expensive anti-ageing moisturiser with SPF. SPF is an all-encompassing product that will overtake any active or expensive ingredients in your skincare. SPF is both chemically and physically a dominating ingredient and if you load a skin cream with it, that's the sole benefit you'll get from the cream. I would never buy an extortionate anti-ageing moisturiser with SPF - you're paying for an expensive SPF. If you can afford it, and you love it, carry on, but you're not getting the best out of your moisturiser. Buy a good moisturiser and a perfectly reasonably priced SPF. Job done.

Acne sufferers: while the sun may have a drying effect on your acne; a lot of SPF products are comedogenic. Use oil-free sunscreens if possible.

SPF degrades. Check for an expiration date, and if it doesn't have one, buy new each year.

WHICH SPF?

If you want proper protection from the sun you need to use a **broad-spectrum sun protectant cream** – a dedicated product that's sole purpose is to protect your skin from the damage the sun does to it.

The round UVA symbol, left, can only be shown on packaging of a product that has been proven to provide at least a third of its protection against UVA. Not just UVB.

Use either SPF30 or 50+, nothing lower.

THE 1 PER CENT

While you may frequently read that there is only around 1 per cent difference between SPF30 and an SPF50 when it comes to UVB exposure, the science clearly shows that there is a huge difference in the cumulative cutaneous UV exposure when using a lower SPF compared to a higher one.

Put simply, the long-term signs of damage on the skin have more chance of being minimised if you consistently use a high SPF.

Be aware of the difference between SPF50 and SPF50+. An SPF50 is tested to be exactly that, but an SPF50+ must achieve at least an SPF 60 to get that '+' sign.

SUN PROTECTION RATINGS

The EU has also reclassified sun protection ratings:

- Low = 6–14
- Medium = 15–29
- High = 30–50
- Very high = 50+

If you are fair, Caucasian or 'pale' you should be in the **'High'** category. If you have a darker skin tone that tans easily and rarely burns you can use **medium** as long as you use it wisely. If you are a redhead, however, you are **strictly in the 'Very high'** category. Redheads with freckles have phaeomelanin – as opposed to the rest of us that have eumelanin. They burn easily and quickly, and the damage will be long-lasting.

When we analyse clients' skin, the main areas that nearly *always* show damage are the tops of the ears (ALWAYS the top of the ears), the back of the neck and the tip of the nose. Forewarned is forearmed.

Enjoy the sun. I LOVE the sun.
Just protect yourself.

HOW MUCH SPF?

Most people apply too little sunscreen. This results in sunscreen users achieving an SPF coverage of 50–80 per cent less than that specified on the product label.[1] You need at least a teaspoonful for each body part – arm, leg (tablespoon for me, thanks!), front, back and face – and don't forget your ears and neck.

Apply 2 milligrams per square centimetre. This equates to approximately:

FACE AND NECK: 2 finger-lengths

CHEST: 2 teaspoons

BACK: 2 teaspoons

ARMS: 2 teaspoons per arm

LEGS: 2–3 teaspoons per leg, depending on your height, obviously

If you are particularly tall, or have a large frame, obviously use more. I use a good two finger-lengths altogether for face, neck and décolleté, but I've got a fat head – and I'm 5'11, so I use 2 tablespoons per body part. Don't be shy!

TRY THESE...

· Ecooking

· EltaMD

· Evy Technology

· Heliocare

· La Roche-Posay Anthelios

· Ultra Violette

GOVERNMENT GUIDELINES

The US's FDA standards and requirements when it comes to SPF formulas and labelling are different from Europe and Australasia. Following these guidelines can make a difference to a sunscreen's effectiveness. Here's how to make sense of it all, and what to look out for.

> In the USA, SPF labelling is a requirement because the FDA says it is a drug.
>
> In Europe, it is classed as a cosmetic and therefore stating SPF classification is not mandatory, it's just for information.

Having said that, European manufacturers are allowed to use seven proven UVA filters while the FDA in the USA only allows three, technically meaning that a European product has the potential to be more effective than an American-made product.

SPF is only relevant to UVB light. PPD, or Persistent Pigment Darkening, is one way of measuring UVA light, but is now considered out-dated. And the PA++ system, developed in Asia, is another method used. However, neither of these are allowed when making broad-spectrum claims in the USA. Still with me? No? I don't blame you. It's beyond confusing for the average consumer.

An in vitro test (see page 254) to gauge a critical wavelength is really what a brand should be able to show in order to claim broad spectrum on their packaging in the US and the UK. Critical wavelength tests measure the absorbance of UV light on skin and a critical wavelength of 370nm is what you are looking for on SPF product literature. Not that many brands will bother labelling that information, so do your research or ask them directly if you are looking for a broad-spectrum product (which I highly recommend).

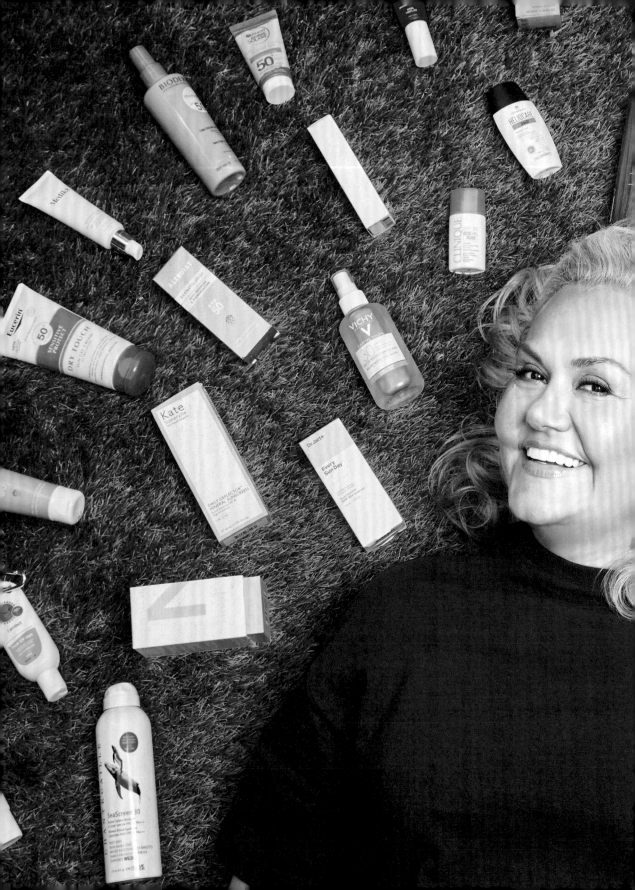

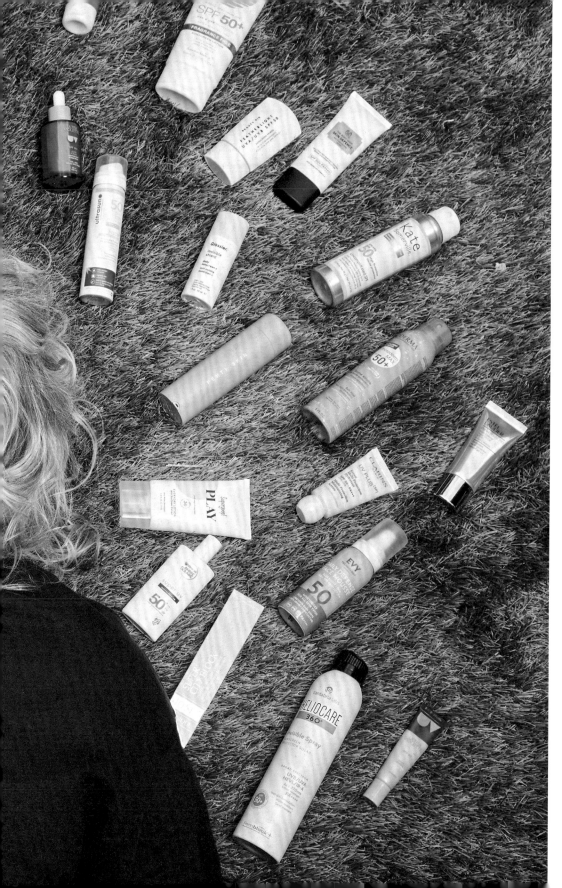

SPF MYTHS

- **'SPF takes 20 minutes to work.'** Not true. The recommendation to apply sunscreen 20 minutes before sun exposure is simply to give it time to spread evenly around your skin. It starts working straight away.

- **'I don't wear SPF as it stops me getting enough vitamin D.'** Categorically untrue. The sun hits the top of your head, your hands, your legs. It's not like your face is the only exposed part of your body.

- **'Mineral SPF is better for pigmentation and melasma.'** Not true.

- **'SPF accumulates.'** Not true. If you wear a moisturiser, primer and sunscreen you will only have the highest SPF that you are using. You cannot 'add them up'.

- **'Sunscreens can be waterproof.'** Not true. No sunscreen is waterproof. They can now only be legally listed as 'water resistant'.

- **'Darker skin tones don't need SPF.'** Absolutely not true. While darker skin tones are not as vulnerable to UV light because of their built-in SPF of around 13.3, they still need protection from UV damage and should use a minimum of SPF30.

- **'I don't need SPF in the car.'** Not true. The sun penetrates glass.

'Pre-cancerous' moles. They are either cancerous or they are not. If in doubt, cut it out. A mole is a benign lesion. If you notice any changes – any – get them checked by an expert.

- **'SPF60 is twice as effective as SPF30.'** Not true. As we've said, while there may only be a 1 per cent difference between SPF30 and SPF50 in theory, there is shown to be a much larger **cumulative cutaneous** UV protection when using a 50. Use SPF50 wherever possible.

- **'Our SPF is Cruelty-Free.'** Not true *in theory*. Never were more ingredients tested on animals in the skincare industry than those that are used in SPF products. This *does not* mean the final product is tested on animals, so brands that state they are against animal testing and say their products are cruelty-free are not technically *lying*. It means the raw ingredients were, at some point, absolutely tested on animals in a lab to ensure 'efficacy', especially in the USA, where they are classed as drugs. This is true of the entire skincare and health industry, and I mention it not to make you feel bad, just purely to counterbalance the rubbish of 'vegan, animal-friendly, non-toxic SPF50' claims that are, frankly, nonsense. PETA can say there are a wealth of cruelty-free brands, but the reality is that the ingredients were tested on animals at some point. They may be cruelty-free now, but the *ingredients* have probably been tested on animals historically.

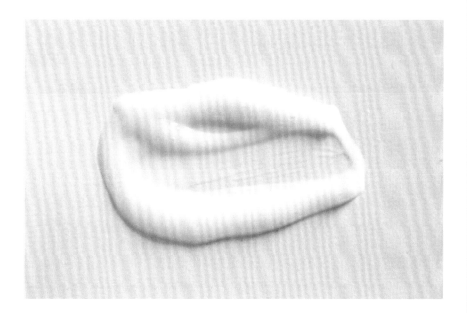

SPF: MY MOST-ASKED QUESTIONS FROM READERS

- **Do 'once-a-day' sunscreens work?**
Personally, I would not dream of using a 'once-a-day' sunscreen on holiday, *especially* on my children. It gives a false sense of security. According to some once-a-day SPF websites, if I use their SPF50 with my skin type, I can 'safely' stay in the sun for ten hours. TEN. HOURS? No. Where once-a-day formulas *might* come in handy are...

Young children going to school. If, as mine did, your young children attend a school where the teachers are not allowed to touch the children, even with your permission, a once-a-day formula may be a good option. Your children may sweat a little, but they aren't in the sea so should still be protected until the end of the day. In *theory*. It makes me uneasy nonetheless, but it's better than applying a typical 'kids' SPF15 first thing and that's it for the day... It's your judgement call as a parent or carer. Remember the backs of their necks and the tops of their ears.

If you are wearing SPF under your makeup and going to work.
You will probably not be covered by lunchtime so you either need to reapply (not likely, I know), use a once-a-day product – these are far better suited to city living than beach in my opinion – or buy yourself a big hat and be done with it.

- **Do you recommend sunscreen sprays?**
  Here's the thing with sprays: they absolutely have their place, but you have to make sure you have covered the entire area thoroughly and that is unlikely unless you are applying it to your child, in which case most of us show more due diligence than when we are applying to our own bodies. You *must* always shake a spray well before use. Use a spray over your makeup if you know you have applied it evenly and feel protected, otherwise, go down the once-a-day route or make like Jackie O and enjoy a hat and sunglasses. There is also cause for concern when inhaling sprays – something you will invariably do if the point is to apply it over your makeup. Your judgement call.

- **Is it safe to use acids and vitamin A products in the summer?**
  Yes absolutely. Just make sure you are using your SPF and you're good to go.

- **Do I need to apply SPF when it's cloudy?**
  Yes. If you can read without an artificial light, you should be wearing SPF.

- **Do I need to reapply if I'm in my office all day?**
  If you go to work in the dark, don't go out for lunch, don't sit near a window and go home in the dark, I'll let you off. If, however, you are out and about in daylight at any point, wear SPF.

It takes 21 days to develop a habit. Set an alarm every morning reminding you to wear SPF. Get into the habit so that it becomes second nature.

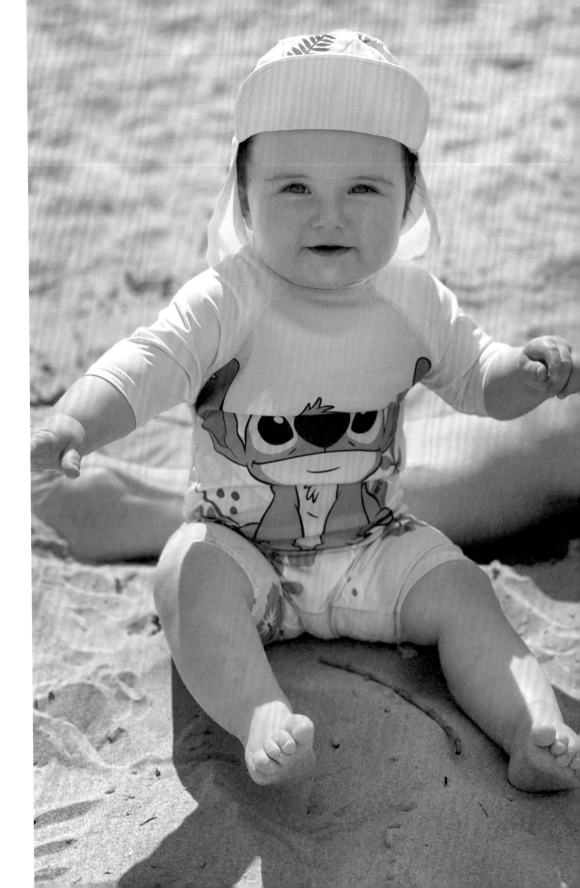

CHILDREN AND SPF

If you have children, the best advice is to cover them up and keep them out of direct sunlight as much as possible.

- General medical advice for babies is to keep them out of the sun and covered up during infancy, and then to use SPF from 6 months old.

- Reapply their SPF every 90 minutes, more frequently if they are getting wet.

- If you have children with short hair, remember to apply sunscreen to the back of their necks and their ears. Every single person I have seen under a Wood's Lamp has significant sun damage at the tops of their ears.

If you or your child have long hair, remember to put your hair up before you apply your SPF. That way you will not forget to protect your ears and the back of your neck.

WHERE SHOULD I SPEND MOST OF MY MONEY?

The answer is always, always serums. Unless you're on a tighter budget, in which case, spend your money on SPF.

The rise of serums has definitely, in my opinion, bumped moisturisers off the top spot, although moisturisers were never my No.1, more the prevailing thought of the industry back in the early days of Estée Lauder and Elizabeth Arden.

> Spend your money on skincare, foundation and concealer and if you want to, use budget for everything else. You will look fabulous.

Spend up to around £150 (outside the organic market) and you will generally **get what you pay for** (in some circumstances you still need to check the ingredients to see what you are paying for). After that, you're paying for packaging, the perceived 'prestige' of using that brand, and the rent, payroll and holiday home of the name on the box.

I fully understand that the majority of us are on much smaller budgets, but if you can, look at the £40–£100 mark for serums if you want them to be hi-tech and include a decent level of active ingredients.

Cleansers can be much more affordable. The Ordinary Squalane Cleanser is one of my favourites and it starts at £5.50. It would have to be a bloody good cleanser or a much larger size to get me to £60. If you want good-quality skincare and are willing to forgo the hi-tech, you can get amazing quality natural or organic products that are more affordable.

I have purposefully not included international prices here because, especially since the effects of Brexit have started to kick in and be felt by brands and suppliers, they are so changeable.

But be aware that the further away you are from a brand's country of origin, the more you will be charged for their product. This unfortunately particularly impacts our friends in the southern hemisphere i.e. Australia and New Zealand.

Ultimately, buy what you can afford and want to spend. Don't credit-card your skincare.

TRY THESE...

Budget Skincare

The following brands are where you will find some good products at an affordable price. While I cannot vouch for every product within every range, you will undoubtedly find some gems, especially when it comes to your basics.

- AVEENO®
- Avène
- Balance Me™
- Boots own label
- BYBI
- Carbon Theory
- CeraVe
- Curél
- e.l.f
- Embryolisse
- Florena
- Garden Of Wisdom

- Hada Labo Tokyo™
- L'Oréal Paris skincare
- La Roche-Posay
- Neutrogena®
- O'Keeffe's
- Palmer's®
- Pixi
- Revolution Beauty skincare
- Simple
- Superdrug own label
- Super Facialist

- Supergoop!
- The INKEY List
- The Ordinary
- Trader Joe's skincare own brand
- UpCircle
- Versed Skincare
- Vichy
- Weleda
- Yes To
- YourGoodSkin

"

THERE IS NOTHING IN YOUR LARDER THAT CAN CURE ACNE. I WISH THERE WAS!

"

HOMEMADE PRODUCTS

Despite what you might read on certain websites, you will find no substitute for good professional skincare in your kitchen. It's wishful thinking. Please do not believe the hype.

The best you can hope for is a temporary softening of the skin (avocado/plain yoghurt) or a very temporary tightening (egg white). The aloe vera that you see listed on a product's INCI list is a world apart from the sticky, clear gel that you get when you cut an aloe leaf. It has to go through a chemical process to even begin to think about penetrating the skin.

There is nothing, I repeat, NOTHING in your larder that can cure acne. I wish there was! But coconut oil, lemon, baking soda, turmeric and the rest all belong in your food, not on your face.

And don't get me started on lemon juice.

'Adding lemon juice to your cleanser will exfoliate your skin!' No, it won't. 'Applying lemon juice to your skin will fix your pigmentation!' No, it won't.

Eat it, by all means.
Just don't add it to any product.

Case in point: anyone remember Sun-In from the 80s? Lots of brunette girls going around with orange hair. Nice.

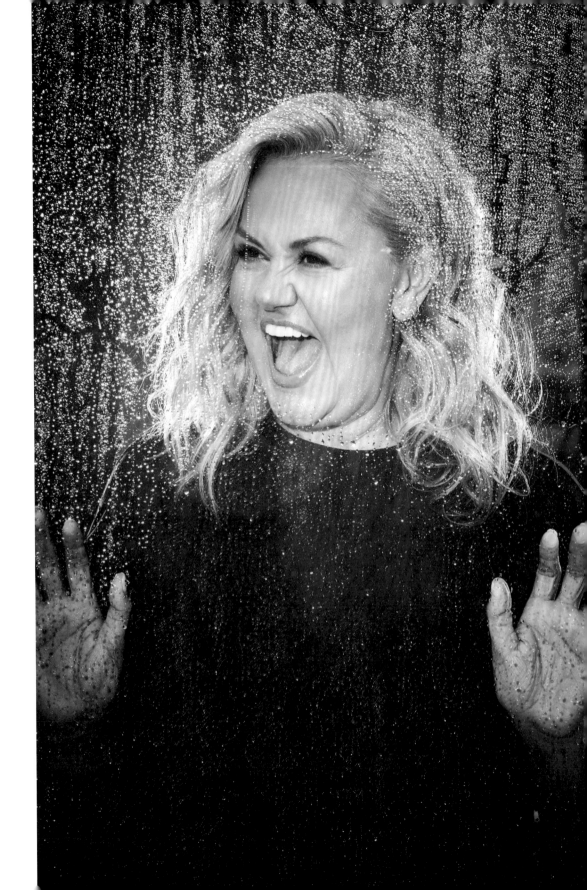

FESTIVAL SKINCARE

This was one of my most popular blog posts, so I'm bringing it out again for all those of you who *will* insist on sleeping in a tent in the pouring rain, drinking yourselves into oblivion and having, at best, questionable hygiene habits for the duration. This, we call 'entertainment'. Personally, I prefer a day ticket, VIP pass and a nice hotel with hot showers, but that's me. God knows what posesses you.

So, you're packed and ready for Glastonbury/Reading/Leeds/Download (me)/Coachella Festival etc. – what's in your skincare stash?

If you're the type of person that keeps their wits about them, you can do most of your normal routine. If, however, you know you're going to party non-stop for 3/4/5 days, I would just take wipes and SPF and deal with the carnage when you get home. At least you'll have a great time without adding sunburn into the mix.

WIPES

If you're going to use a wipe, now is the time. Bear in mind, like good tea and 80s rock bands, all wipes are not created equal (see 'Try These...' on page 172).

However: if you can, I'd go with a **micellar water/eye-makeup remover and cotton-wool pads**. They just do a better job.

I also love a good traditional milk cleanser in this situation, one that can either be washed off in the shower (literally going against my religion here, I know) or removed with cotton pads.

But still, if you're boozing, stick to wipes. And have the foresight to take two packets: one to keep in your bag (PortaKabin toilet horror) and one to leave in your tent/accommodation to remove your makeup.

Pictured left: Your average festival weather in the UK.

ACID

Here's the thing. I would probably not bother with acid during the day at a festival. You're going to be outside all day, sitting in the sun (although if you're in the sun, you're probably not in the UK), you may be drunk/tipsy and forget to apply your SPF... is it worth it?

For the sake of 3 days, give it a miss. If, however, you're going for longer and want to use acids to 'back up' your wipes, use them in the evening and make sure you have your SPF for the next day. Ready-soaked acid pads are an obvious choice here.

Failing that, pre-soak your own cotton pads in your chosen acid toner and put them in a Ziplock lunch bag. It's what I used on flights before they made pre-soaked pads...

If you have time, can be bothered, and know you will use it, I would take some La Roche-Posay Serozinc with you. This face toner mist may help keep your skin hydrated, can be used to help remove wipe residue and is antibacterial. It also comes in a travel size. Well handy.

SERUM

There's really only one choice for festival serum and that's hyaluronic acid. You need it. Whether you're boozing or not, the weather (sun, wind or rain) will take its toll on your hydration levels, so the easiest way to keep it topped up is with a dose of hyaluronic acid. This is not the time for your expensive anti-ageing serums. Save your money.

My first choice would be a hyaluronic acid product in a plastic tube (avoid fiddly packaging or glass containers – not what you want in a tent or, God forbid, a shared cubicle shower monstrosity). You could also use a hydrating spray or hyaluronic acid mist.

MOISTURISERS

For ease, if you have to, use one with SPF included. For safety, I'd personally use a good hydrating moisturiser and a high, broad-spectrum SPF on top. If you can take your normal moisturiser and it's not in any heavy/glass packaging, do. Tubes and pumps are obviously safer and more hygienic.

"

WIPES ARE FOR FANNIES, FLIGHTS AND FESTIVALS ONLY

"

SPF

Take SPF50. Don't faff about with an SPF15 – it's pointless, especially in this scenario. Apply a cream to your face and body in the morning and carry a spray to top up throughout the day. For more on SPF, see pages 146–163.

WHERE TO DO IT ALL IN A ROUTINE

Assuming you're doing the festival in a fairly controlled manner and get up and go to the showers at a decent hour in the morning, cleanse with your micellar water or milk cleanser and flannel if you can (please). Make sure your skin is as clean as you can get it, apply your hyaluronic acid and your moisturiser, then your SPF. I know for a lot of you this will be your only cleanse of the day that goes anywhere near water.

If, in the evenings, you get back to your tent a little worse for wear and manage to wipe your face down a few times and apply a moisturiser on top, well done.

If you *can*, use your wipes or micellar water, then serum, then moisturiser. Just do your best. Let's face it, the point of a festival is not meticulous skincare.

TRY THESE...

- Clinique Take The Day Off Face and Eye Cleansing Towelettes
- Curél Deep Moisture Spray
- Glossier Milky Jelly Cleanser
- La Roche-Posay Anthelios SPF50
- La Roche-Posay Serozinc Face Toner Mist
- NIOD Multi-Molecular Hyaluronic Complex MMCH2
- REN Perfect Canvas Clean Jelly Oil Cleanser
- The Body Shop Camomile Gentle Eye Make-Up Remover
- The Ordinary Natural Moisturising Factors + HA
- Then I Met You Living Cleansing Balm
- Ultrasun (they specialise in once a day application)
- Ultra Violette (any)

CELEBS DON'T WASH THEIR FACES

Here's the thing: if you don't want to use anything on your skin, don't. If you want to only use mānuka honey on your skin, do. If you don't want to wash your face ever, that's up to you.

The 'caveman' regimen trend has been aided and abetted by reports of certain celebrities who swear they 'only ever use soap and water' on their skin and are 'horrified' at the thought of washing their faces in the mornings.

Firstly, let's be clear. Celebrities telling us they don't wash their faces and saying they only use soap and water is not new. Some have always said that. It was utter bollocks then, and it is now.

The 'average' woman (you and me) feels enough pressure to be perfect without XYZ celeb saying they don't work out (lies), they eat 'everything in sight!' (lies) and now that they don't wash their face at all? Give me a motherflannel-loving break.

If it was just celebs being arses it wouldn't be that big of a deal, but there is a whole industry behind this caveman crapola. You can spend a lot of hard-earned cash to be shown how NOT to use any products on your skin.

pauses

Yes, of course you can use too much stuff on your face. I've always said do what you have to do for you – whatever that is. But please don't think that these people have perfect skin without skincare and/or without medical intervention. The jig is up, people. Enough.

Now, go wash your faces.

UP IN THE AIR: SKINCARE WHEN TRAVELLING

I travel a lot and take more than my fair share of long-haul flights. I always travel makeup free, covered in skincare products, and I have my in-air kit down to a fine art:

- **Tissues or wipes,** or both. I always need a small packet of tissues and I use face wipes on planes too, but mainly for my hands. I can't remember the last time I used a wipe on my face.

- **Hand sanitiser.** A no-brainer. If you're applying product to your face, your hands need to be clean, and when you're on a plane, there's not always a convenient time/place to wash them.

- **Hand cream or medicated/antibacterial cream.** Putting some hand cream just inside your nostrils when you're on the go – especially when flying – is a well-known travelling tip. The air on the plane is recirculated and really dehydrating to your skin, and the theory is that when your nasal hair is dried out it offers no protection against airborne germs. I used to always get sick after flying – usually getting a sore throat for a few days – but then I started doing the hand cream trick and it worked. Any hand cream will work.

- A small, refillable, plastic spray bottle from Muji filled with a **hyaluronic acid or glycerin-based mist.** I probably use this more than anything else.

- **Eye drops.** I haven't always travelled with eye drops and I don't know why. They're great for dry eyes, itchy eyes and again, help keep the warm, damp areas on the face from drying out. They are obviously totally optional, but I now take them on every flight.

- **Eye product.** Not vital, but I get dry eyes when I travel and I wear glasses. I am never more than 3 feet from my eye cream on a normal day, never mind in a dried-out, airless vacuum.

- **Facial oil.** I usually use a plain squalane oil, but you could use whatever your skin loves. My skin loves squalane. I can use it to calm it down, or to give it a layer of protection, applying it after or before other actives or serums (depending on the action of the other product), and it is hands-down one of my favourite facial oils ever. It works well under or over pretty much any product.

- **Moisturiser.** Which you use depends on your skin type (see pages 65–66). I like a hydrating emulsion as opposed to a thick occlusive cream.

- **SPF.** If you're travelling in daylight and sitting near the window, don't forget your SPF.

- **Lip balm.** The lips are usually the first area of the face to dry out, especially on a flight. I love a hybrid between a lip balm and a gloss; this saves me carrying two separate items.

TRY THESE...

- Biossance 100% Squalane Oil
- Kopari Coconut Lip Glossy
- Lanolips Face Base The Aussie Jetlag Face Mask
- La Roche-Posay Toleriane Ultra 8
- Nivea Biodegradable Cleansing Wipes

- O'Keeffe's Working Hands Hand Cream
- Ole Henriksen Truth On The Glow™ Cleansing Cloths
- REN Vita Mineral™ Omega 3 Optimum Skin Oil
- The Body Shop Camomile Gentle Eye Make Up Remover

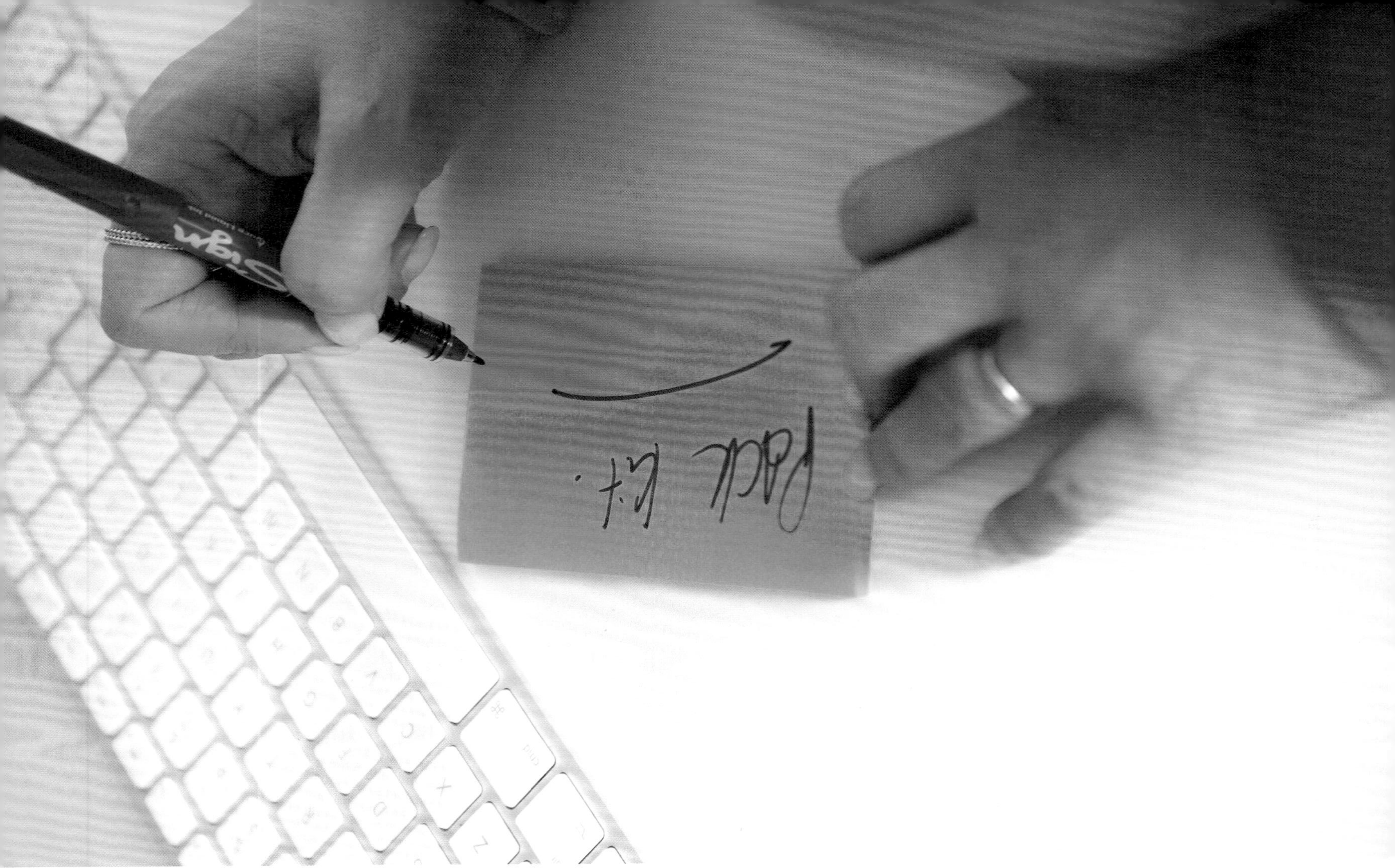
Pack kit.

SUMMER SKIN

Sometimes the first warm day of spring or summer sneaks up on you and you find your makeup feels heavy, or your creams suddenly feel sticky.

The change from cold to warm, from using central heating to sitting in an air-conditioned office, means you need to make a few simple swap-outs to your routine. You will still be layering your skincare, but using less of your topical product and/or switching out a couple of key products for lighter options.

FIVE THINGS TO CHANGE FOR SUMMER

Here are five key things to consider changing in your skincare routine when you pack away your winter woollies.

#1 CLEANSING

Cleansing milks and gels are light and won't feel heavy in the heat. I use balms all year round, but I know a younger, more combination skin frequently finds them a tad heavy.

#2 SPF AND SUNBURN

As the days get longer, don't forget to up the ante on your SPF. If you enjoy sitting out in the summer evenings, and you last applied your SPF when you left for work, it's worth carrying a spray or mineral SPF so you can top-up throughout the day (neither are perfect for coverage, so just do your best). Don't go lower than an SPF30.

There is no such thing as a 'safe' tan. If you do get sunburned, strip back actives, take down the heat and keep the skin cool with regular cold showers and wet cloths. Take aspirin or ibuprofen and wear loose clothing that protects the burned areas.

"

THERE IS NO SUCH THING AS A SAFE TAN

"

#3 ACIDS AND SERUMS

Glycolic acid does make you more sensitive to the sun, however, it doesn't stop me recommending it or using it myself. Just make sure you are using your SPF.

In all its forms, hyaluronic acid (HA) is great for hot weather as long as you are using it alongside something else, whether it's a moisture-loaded mist or a light moisturiser. Some hyaluronic serums are actually hybrid moisturisers, if you are using a serum or a very light moisturiser that contains a good dose of HA, you may find it's enough.

#4 ANTIOXIDANTS

Vitamin C is a powerful antioxidant that helps protect against free radicals and encourages collagen production. It is of course recommended year-round, but it's worth another mention for the warmer months. You'll probably be outside more, in sunlight for longer, and who doesn't like the added glow?

#5 MOISTURISER

Oil-free moisturiser is obviously an option for oilier skins year-round, but it becomes a good option for the rest of us in higher temperatures. Your skin will be able to retain more of its own moisture in humidity, so if your products feel a little heavy, or greasy, switch to a lighter, and perhaps oil-free, moisturiser until the weather cools down.

DON'T SCRIMP ON SPF

If you are sitting in the sun, you need to reapply sunscreen every 2 hours, no matter the factor.

- Apply your SPF 15–20 minutes before you go in the sun to allow it to spread on your skn evenly.

- Reapply SPF every 90 minutes to 2 hours, or more often if in water.

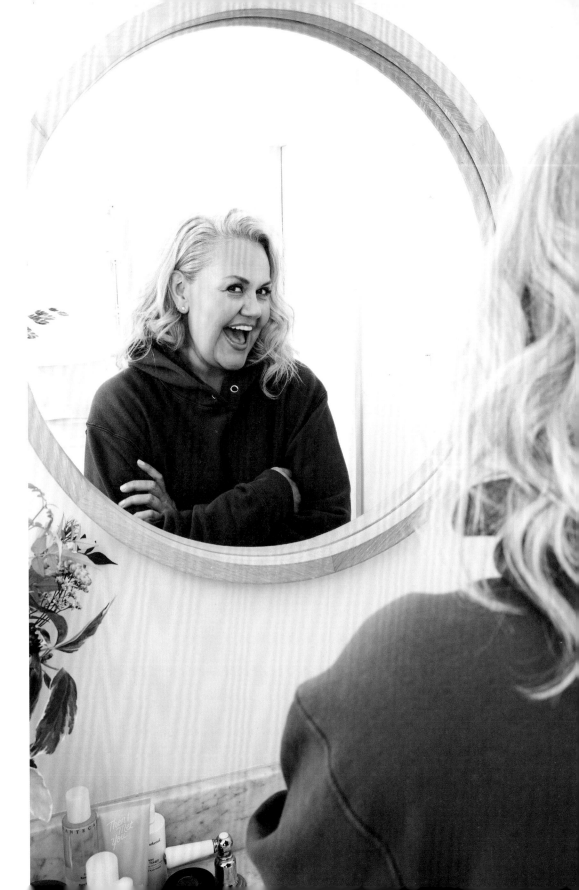

WINTER SKIN

The change from warm to cold, from central heating to cold, can really make your skin feel parched.

Here are a few tips that may help keep your skin feeling hydrated, plump and healthy.

- Treat the skin like you do your clothing. If you're layering clothing, **layer your skincare**. You need a skincare 'wardrobe' at this time of year more than any other. Cleanse, tone (acid/mist or both), serum, oil, cream, SPF and/or balm. How much and when you use all of these depends on your skin, but a general rule of thumb is to start with 'less is more' and if your skin is still absorbing the product, **keep going** (the only thing to be aware of is layering silicone products, as they don't always play well together and have the potential to 'peel' or 'roll', which feels grim).

- **Don't over-cleanse.** Your skin needs all the moisture it can get at this time of year. If your skin is dry/sensitive and you are using harsh cleansers suitable for the summer months, or even worse, overusing the electronic facial cleansing brushes (see pages 268–270), it may be very unforgiving.

- **Avoid alcohol-heavy products.** It's one thing to have a toner with *alcohol denat* at the very end of the INCI list (see Glossary), but it's another to have alcohol as the main ingredient. Acids can be an exception here, as alcohol is used to stabilise the formula.

- If you love an old-school foaming face wash, consider **changing to a cleansing milk** if your skin feels drier when the weather is cold. You can buy a milk for oily skin if you need it.

- **Oils and balms** can feel very comforting on the skin. Natural ones. If your skin is particularly dry, a heavy balm may actually be stripping it, so go easy. For oily skin, use an oil designed for its specific type.

- You should **NEVER** aim for 'squeaky clean' on any part of your body, be it hair or skin. If you have this feeling after washing/cleansing, you really need to **stop and rethink** what you are using.

- **Exfoliate** your face and body regularly. Topical exfoliants in liquid form are far more effective than scrubs. Skin is acidic and it is receptive to acid products. Use toners or pads with AHA acids (see Glossary) twice a day and follow with a spray of a hydrating toner containing glycerin and/or hyaluronic acid before you apply your serum and you'll feel a difference after one day.

- Not everyone can use/wants to use liquid acids. For those of you that prefer a physical exfoliant, aim for gentle, naturally sourced granular scrubs that don't use beads. The ones that dissolve as you are rubbing them in are generally safest.

- Ensure you are taking **omega oils** to help your skin internally. Fish oils are the best – flax are a good second for vegetarians and vegans.

- Do continue to use face masks, but go for more **hydrating** ones as opposed to clay ones. If you have a combination skin, use your clay mask and go straight in afterwards with a hydrating one for a good boost.

- If you are a shower person, **do not** be tempted to stand under a hot shower to warm up. Your skin will not thank you for it. Keep it warm-hot, not boiling!

- If you suffer from psoriasis (see page 72) or eczema (see page 70) it is likely that you will experience a worsening of symptoms in the colder months. Make sure your shower/bath products are as irritant-free as possible, **avoid** tumble dryer sheets as they can also aggravate the skin, and remember to **moisturise.**

- And finally: **do not forget your vitamin D**. You can buy vitamin D supplements either as a spray or as tablets, though as with all supplements, always follow your doctor's advice.

"MOISTURISE, MOISTURISE, MOISTURISE!!!"

VITAMIN D

Vitamin D is crucial for your overall health. I tell anyone who will listen about all number of supplements, but vitamin D has been my obsession for a while.

Too much sun can be bad for you – *really* bad for you. So, too, can *too little* sun. Particularly in the northern hemisphere, where most people living modern life spend a larger proportion of their time indoors, and with most of their skin surface covered by clothing or sunscreen when outdoors, there is a growing deficiency in vitamin D. Vitamin D needs to be present in your system for the intestines to absorb dietary calcium.

Vitamin D is actually, in its truest form, a hormone, and it is essential for our wellbeing, yet the use of sunscreens prevents the development of vitamin D in the body. Vitamin D also degrades as quickly as it generates, creating another stumbling block to retaining it in our system.

- **Vitamin D can reduce your risk of the flu and health complications related to flu.** Vitamin D contributes to lowering the incidence of infections and inflammation during the autumn–winter flu season. The Canadian government has recommended increased vitamin D intake as part of their flu prevention strategy, including prevention of swine flu.[2]

- **Vitamin D can help reduce your risk of depression.**[3]

- **Vitamin D can reduce chronic muscle aches and pain.** Vitamin D helps to normalise blood calcium, which is required in order for tight, shortened muscles to soften, lengthen and relax out of spasm.

- **Vitamin D can reduce your risk of cancer.** Low levels of vitamin D are associated with an increased incidence of many cancers.[4]

- **Vitamin D can reduce your risk of developing Type 1 diabetes.**[5]

According to NHS guidelines,[6] everyone (including pregnant and breastfeeding women) should consider taking a daily supplement containing 10 micrograms of vitamin D during the autumn and winter.

People with darker skin tones make less vitamin D than those with paler skin.

Ageing skin makes 75 per cent less vitamin D than young skin.

Vitamin D-rich foods include cold-water fish such as wild salmon, wild cod and sardines and cod liver oil. However, you would need to eat mammoth amounts of these foods to build up your vitamin D stores. If you're shopping for supplements, look for vitamin D3 listed on the label.

FIVE THINGS TO CHANGE FOR WINTER

Here are a few key things to consider changing in your skincare routine when you swap your rain mac for something woolly!

#1 CLEANSING

If you worship at the altar of wipes and harsher foaming cleansers, you might find your skin slightly more unforgiving in a colder climate. Switch to milks, creams and balms and you'll feel a difference in your skin at once.

#2 TONERS

Keep up with the acids. Now is not the time to slow down. Acids are crucial for keeping your skin exfoliated and fresh, and ready to accept anything that follows them. Treat yourself to a new one and keep the skin challenged in a safe, non-aggressive way. If you can afford it, absolutely use more than one.

#3 FACIAL OILS

If you don't already use one, now is the time to consider investing. If you've already boarded the facial oil train, try two drops under your moisturiser in the mornings to keep your skin protected throughout the day. Skin shouldn't feel greasy when you do this; if it does, you're using too much product. Remember: **Grip, not slip.**

#4 CHANGE YOUR ROUTINE TIMES

Take advantage of the darker nights and perhaps getting home earlier and do your routine as soon as you get in from work/school run/college. Full cleanse, acid, serum/oil application. Go about your business, check your skin hourly until you go to bed, and reapply if you feel like your skin is still absorbing. The skin has done most of its repairing work by 11pm, so don't leave it until 10.30pm when you're going to bed – give it as much time as possible.

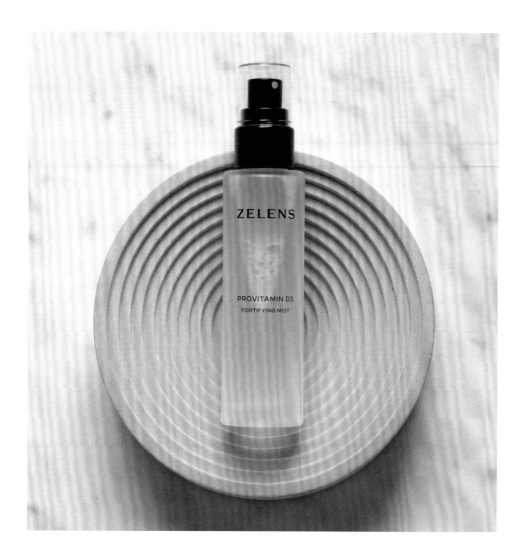

#5 UPGRADE YOUR SPRITZES OR ESSENCES AND USE THEM LIBERALLY

This is no time to be using spray water, like Evian in a can. You'll be dehydrated already and that will just make it worse. Use spritzes or essences that contain other ingredients, like minerals and oils. They work as an extra layer of hydration and hold everything that follows in place, including individual serums and oils.

FACE WIPE FIENDS: If all else fails, cleanse with a balm, remove with a flannel, then apply acid and oil. **That** is your bare minimum, not a wipe.

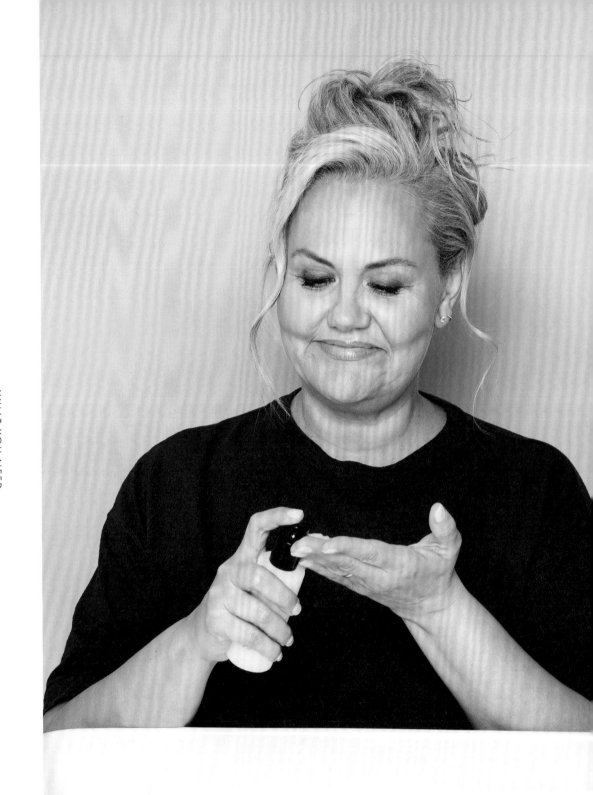

TREATMENTS

It is worth mentioning that although a good skincare routine will undoubtedly improve the quality of your skin, glowing, clear skin is different to facial structure. No amount of skincare will actually stop you ageing or change the *structure* of your skin. If you are more concerned about the signs of ageing such as a heavy brow, hollow cheeks, sagging jawline or hooded eyelids, you'll need either a needle or an operation. To be clear, I am not suggesting for one second that you actually *need* any interventions with your face; I am merely trying to manage expectations.

It would also be helpful to change the conversation around things like Botox and filler in the media. Saying things like 'of course they've got good skin, they've had Botox/filler' etc. is just not scientifically correct. Every time I speak to people in the media, they say, 'What have you had done?' as if that negates years of a good skin routine. Yes, I've had filler twice (see overleaf), and will definitely have it again at some point, and I've had my eyelids done – they were so heavy that they were impairing my vision (I would highly recommend this if you are in a similar boat) – but I've also looked after my skin.

Botox and filler change the *structure* of your skin, not the *surface* of it. You may have plumper, higher cheeks, but you could still have acne, pigmentation, redness, dryness and the other conditions discussed in this book. That's where good skincare comes in. Having said that, sometimes you can have a good skincare routine and use the right products, but your skin either does not respond, it has a bigger issue that requires professional or medical intervention, or is simply showing natural signs of ageing.

COMMON COMPLAINTS

Outside of specific skin complaints, such as acne or dermatitis, the following signs of ageing are what often bring people to the clinic door, whether it be for treatments with a facialist or more invasive options with a dermatologist or qualified doctor:

- More obvious lines on the face that do not improve when your usual products or topicals are applied.

- Skin is noticeably less firm as you move closer to, and through, menopause (see page 209).

- Pigmentation (see page 71): whether related to the condition known as melasma, post-inflammatory pigmentation or good old sun damage, this is an issue I am often asked about at my events and on my social media accounts.

- The fat pads in your cheek area shrink with age, giving you not so much a thinner face, more of a gaunt one.

- Sagging skin: this is caused by the ageing process and those fat pads in your cheeks diminishing.

- Dry, dull skin: this is a result of your inability to retain oil and water in the surface of the skin, and it can make your skin look 'flat' and lifeless. There is very little moisture in the skin to reflect the light.

- Alongside your cheek pads, bone recedes, most noticeably around the eye and brow area, causing the sunken appearance of older eyes.

- Broken capillaries or thread veins: general (and very common) signs of wear and tear on the skin.

'TWEAKMENTS'

In my 'Skincare Freaks' Facebook group, people post a lot of pictures pre- and post- treatment. They want to hear what others think, which is fine, but at the end of the day, the fact is that you should only do this for you. And if you see pictures of someone else after a treatment, don't just say they looked better before. Either pay them a compliment or, as I love to say, get in the sea.

If you **do** feel like you want 'more', at what age should you delve into having treatments that go further than an over-the-counter serum or cream, and a standard 'facial'? This depends very much on your genes and lifestyle.

The goal is a healthy skin, not to make you look permanently surprised.

Ageing is a privilege not everyone gets.

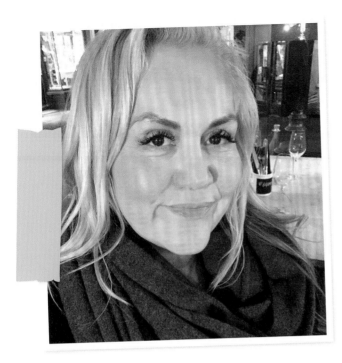

Me after my first round of a small amount of cheek filler.

If you are interested in having some slightly more invasive treatments, or are interested in what is possible with aesthetics, I highly recommend the book *The Tweakments Guide* by Alice Hart-Davis. Alice goes into the minutiae of what to expect, what to look out for, everything that is available on the market and how to find not only a treatment plan for you, but all-round best practice. As an aside, I think Alice's book is also an absolute must for any fellow beauty therapists out there. The book has an accompanying website with a 'tweakment finder tool'.

In the meantime, if you have good skin and are happy with it, excellent. If you are not happy with your skin, use the lists on the next two pages as a rough guide. They are not intended as a timetable or instructions, just a helping hand if you're finding the products you use in your daily routine aren't giving you the results you desire. I've arranged them by age, as 'tweakments' vary in strength and skin suitability.

Firstly, let us not discount the traditional machinery used in various types of facials that is still relevant and suitable for most ages and skins. Faradic and microcurrent (its newer version), galvanic, high-frequency, radio-frequency (see Glossary) — all of these treatments have led to more sophisticated options that are now available to all, such as laser, botox, fillers, PRP, ultherapy and thread lift.

20s:

- Prevention is always better than cure, so please don't stop using SPF. You won't see it now, but you'll be saving yourself a lot of time and effort when you're in your 40s and signs of sun damage start to show through.

- Facials can help with extractions, gentle resurfacing and longer-term issues such as light, fresh scarring and problem complexions.

- Light peels will help manage combination skins and are not contraindicated at any age. Salicylic or lactic acid are great at this age.

- If you have genetic lines on your skin that bother you at this stage, you might consider some superficial or 'baby' botox to help the lines from becoming static. Please only go to reputable derms/qualified practitioners for this – do not ever be tempted by botox 'parties', ever.

30s:

- Pigmentation caused by sun damage in your earlier years will start to come through at this age. Fractional laser and microneedling are all options at this point.

- You may appreciate slightly stronger peels in your 30s, and progressing into stronger acids is an option.

- Your forehead and eye area may be showing deeper lines and/or 'crow's feet'. This is the area I am most frequently asked about. Botox will nip this in the bud quickly and without pain (no, genuinely, a pin-prick on your finger is more painful).

40s:

- Your collagen and facial fat starts to deplete in your 40s, and that is impossible to replace without a needle, despite what some brands would have you believe. Well-placed filler will literally replace the structure lost in your face. It is worth remembering that filler merely aids the structure of the face; it does not affect the skin topically.

- Injectable moisture treatments are hugely beneficial at this age and beyond, and practically painless. Two treatments a year are recommended for very visible results.

- Stronger high-percentage peels are excellent for general skin tone, pigmentation issues and late-onset hormonal spots.

50s+:

- Loss of elastin and collagen are most noticeable now, especially during and after menopause. This age group will have the most visible and immediate results from the following treatments:

  Fillers, botox, laser, radio-frequency, PRP, ultherapy, thread lift... the options are endless and limited only to how much you want to tweak and, of course, how much you have to spend.

DERMATOLOGISTS

I am always asked for derm recommendations and when it's the right time to see a dermatologist. Dermatologists are the specialists you want to seek out if...

- You have severe acne (obviously try not to wait until it gets that bad, but if you have it on your face and back, please go down the medical route as a matter of priority).

- You have allergies or dermatitis. You will know if this has happened: your face will be hot, itchy, inflamed and potentially have small pustules. Go to your doctor in the first instance, then a derm if necessary.

- You have unexplained rashes. In the first instance go to your doctor, then depending on how happy you are with the treatment they prescribe, and the outcome, go to a dermatologist.

As with all roles in life, not all 'doctors' or their brands are created equal, or are as straightforward as they appear. Just because a product says 'Dr' on the label does not mean that the person who created it is qualified in dermatology. At the time of writing, basic medical training gives students very little training on the head and facial anatomy – I can't blame them, they have a lot to cover. In the UK, they get just half a day. *Half a day.*

As a potential patient, you need to do your research before visiting someone who may potentially be injecting you, lasering you or operating on you.

Find out:

- Are they specialists in their field?
- Where did they train?
- What level of training in dermatology do they actually have, if any?
- Are they a consultant on the plastic surgeon register?

All this information should be included on their website. As with all things, if their training was good, they'll be shouting about it.

Outside of personal recommendations from someone whose opinion you trust, if you are ever unsure you can visit the General Medical Council's website, click on 'search the register', enter the doctor's name and gender and their registration will be there for you to check. Ideally, you're looking for 'this doctor is on the specialist register' and the 'specialist register entry date' will tell you what their speciality is. Similar registers are available in all countries, and by state in the USA. You may also see 'Registered as a GP with a special interest in dermatology'. There are of course extremely knowledgeable doctors that work in skin who, for whatever reason, did not take the full dermatology training route, but really know their stuff. This is where personal recommendation, reputation and trust comes into play. Do not be afraid to ask for credentials. (For some of my favourite dermatologists, see The Brands section on pages 294–305.)

DOCTORS AND SKIN

Do bear in mind that completing basic medical school means that someone can call themselves a 'doctor' (as can someone with a PhD in any topic). A board-certified dermatologist has been through a further 6–8 years of training, specifically in skin. There are over 3,000 diseases of the skin, and these are not covered in basic medical training. By all means go to qualified doctors and nurses for aesthetics, but I always go to a board-certified dermatologist for actual 'skin' issues.

There is one notable exception to the 'stick to derms' rule for aesthetics, and that is dentists that have moved into aesthetics. Outside of derms, specialised surgeons and ENTs, there are few medical people more well-trained in facial anatomy.

FACIALISTS AND AESTHETICIANS

Thankfully, not everything requires medical intervention, and this is where facialists and aestheticians come in.

As with the medical field, all facialists are not created equal. All qualifications in England are regulated by Ofqual (Office of Qualifications) on behalf of the Department for Education. The most basic level of training in the UK is considered an ITEC/CIBTAC Level 2 (even these vary slightly), which – at the time of writing – requires 390 hours training, 300 of which are under the guidance of a tutor. To become a fully qualified beauty therapist in the UK, the TQT (total qualification time) is 990 hours. After this, there's specialised training, where you will find lasers, IPL (intense pulse light), advanced radio-frequency, dermapen/needling and the like.

There is currently no central register for therapists in the UK, and the industry is still self-regulated. BABTAC (British Association of Beauty Therapy and Cosmetology) offers a directory and insurance to qualified and verified practitioners, but each borough requires individual registering before therapists can work.

Most reputable clinics/treatment rooms will have their licences and insurance certificates displayed prominently in reception.

The USA is different again, with the hours required for qualification varying dramatically across the individual states. Florida, for example, only requires 250 hours of training, whereas Washington requires 750 for your basic aesthetician licence, with a further 450 required for the Master Aesthetician qualification. Some states will allow you to inject under the guidance of a doctor's clinic, but others, like California, won't even let you break the skin with a lancet to remove milia or perform dermaplane on clients. It's a minefield.

You will need to check the qualifications in your home country, so always do your research. Seek recommendations and don't be afraid to ask questions. It's your face!

WHAT FACIAL?

Despite their popularity and the continued growth of spas and salons, the average woman in the UK has a facial as a 'treat' on only three occasions in their lifetime: a birthday, Christmastime/celebration or their wedding.

There is nothing more frustrating than looking forward to something, paying out good money and coming away feeling dissatisfied. Here's a general guide of what's out there and when it might prove useful.

There are lots of different types of facials, yet most involve the following steps:

- Cleanse
- Exfoliation (sometimes with steam)
- Extraction
- Massage
- Mask
- Application of product

TYPES OF FACIAL

MAINTENANCE: Will include massage, extractions, steam and possibly machinery

PAMPERING: Lots of massage, possible steam and lots of masks or serums

CLEANSING: Massage, clay masks, steam and usually extractions

TREATMENT: Machinery such as FRAXEL, fractional laser (all lasers), light therapy, galvanic, Caci, microneedling and serums/massage

ACNE: Deep cleanse, exfoliation, extraction, masks, high-frequency treatment

GETTING MARRIED

You don't want to walk down the aisle on the biggest day of your life with a beetroot face or spots. If you want to gear up for your wedding and your skin needs a little help...

- Try to start around 4 months before – 6 if you can afford it.

- Have a couple of maintenance facials 6 weeks apart, then a pampering facial a couple of days before the big day itself.

- Avoid invasive machinery, extractions and anything you haven't had before on the last facial before the wedding. No 'last-minute' peels!

If the dress of your dreams is backless or low on the back and you're worried about spots on your back, speak to your facialist – they can treat it.

CELEBRATIONS

If you fancy a one-off treat for a special occasion, go for a pampering facial.

- You want something that includes plenty of massage, masks, serums and moisturisers to leave your skin plumped up and bouncy – something that will last for around 48 hours.

- Avoid extractions or *too much* steam, which can leave you red-faced and dehydrated.

- This is not the time to have a go at those spots.

MY FAVOURITE FACIALISTS

- Dija Ayodele (UK)*
- Antonia Burrell (UK)*
- Sean Garrette (US)*
- Abigail James (UK)
- Andy Millward (UK)
- Pamela Marshall (UK)

- Jennifer Rock (Ireland)
- Olga Kochlewska (Ireland)
- Nayamka Roberts-Smith (US)*
- Nerida Joy (US)
- Candice Miele (US)

- Renée Rouleau (US)
- Jordan Samuel (US)
- Kate Somerville (US)
- Teresa Tarmey (US/UK)
- Debbie Thomas (UK)
- Joanna Vargas (US)

*specialises in darker skin tones

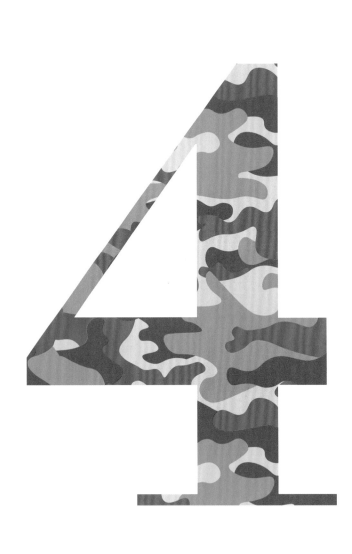

WHEN
LIFE
HAPPENS

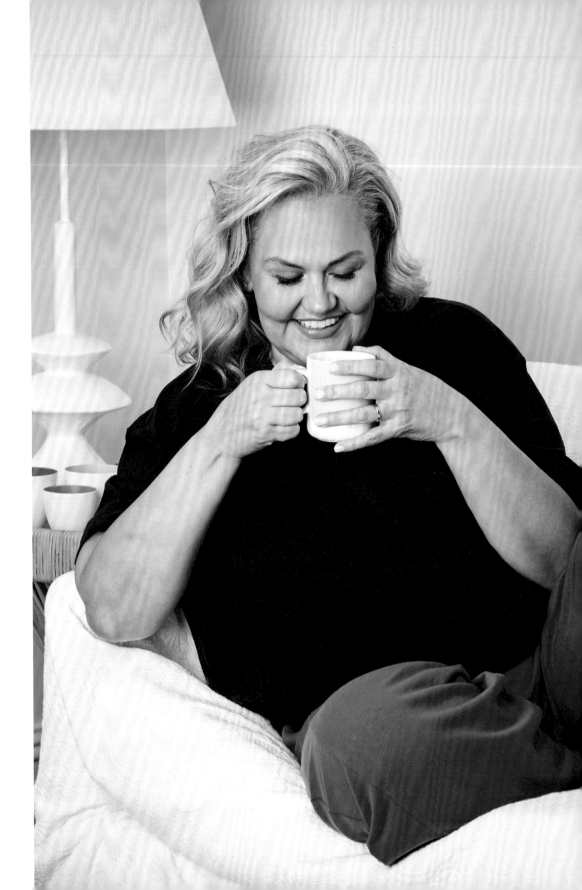

SKIN THROUGH YOUR LIFETIME

▌ Work with your skin, not against it.

As you age, your skin changes, and your skincare routine and kit need to adapt with it.

The best thing you can do for your skin is get into good habits young (wear your SPF, people!), then tackle signs of ageing when you see them – skin starts to lose the ability to retain moisture in the face as you get older, your collagen is depleted and you need to step things up a notch.

Life throws many skin challenges our way, thanks to our hormones, habits, our environment etc. Don't let it blindside you: this section will make sure you're well prepped.

THE THREE WORST THINGS FOR YOUR SKIN

SUN: get a little, not a lot. Be sensible.

SUGAR: probably one of the best (and hardest) things you can do for yourself, your health and your skin is to cut out sugar. In a nutshell, sugar works to destroy your collagen – think of collagen as scaffolding for your face. Every time you eat/drink sugar it is like taking a piece of the scaffolding away – leading to saggy, baggy and drawn skin.

SMOKING: I was once able to tell a client how she blew her smoke out of her mouth (straight up her face from her bottom lip) because of the condition of her skin in the middle panel of her face. Smoking leaches the oxygen out of your face with every puff. Smokers have grey skin. If you smoke, try to get help and stop, as soon as you can.

THE AGEING TRIANGLE

Getting older should be seen as a privilege, not a problem. Some people don't get to see their 40th, 60th or 80th birthdays. Rather than whinging about ageing, let's be grateful that we're still here.

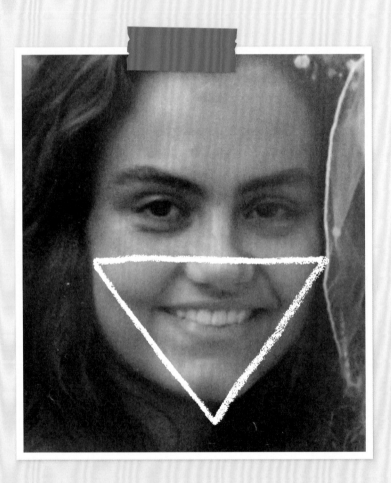

This photo was taken when I was in my early 20s, before my collagen decided to go on holiday. As you can see, all the definition is in the middle of my face. I have solid, high cheekbones, fat cheek pads and very few lines. My eyelids are not hooded and the area under the eye is full.

As you age, your face shape changes. The production of collagen in your skin decreases rapidly after 30. You can think about this like a triangle shape in the bottom half of your face. When you're younger, the base of the triangle is at the top, with the definition at the two corners of your cheekbones, moving to a point at your chin. As you age, the definition – the base of the triangle – moves towards your jawline with the point at your nose. So, the products you're applying need to go from protecting to repairing and supporting.

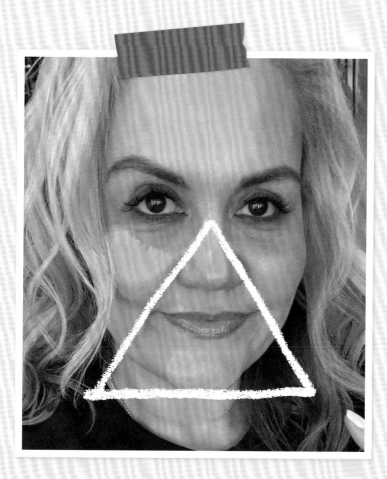

This photo is me in my 40s. The definition has all fallen towards my jawline. The collagen in my skin is massively depleted, therefore the structure of my skin has naturally altered. No amount of product will lift that cheek pad, no matter what the marketing on the packet says. The only thing that will lift this is a needle.

> Hormones are potentially the biggest skin disruptor of all.

Hormones, hormones, hormones. They have a lot to answer for, and at certain times of our lives they RAGE. When this happens, and when illness happens, there are things you can do to help tackle the effects they have on the skin. It just takes a few tweaks to your kit.

PUBERTY

WHAT HAPPENS?

Poor teenagers. Just as your hormones erupt, so do your moods and in some cases, so does your skin. When children go through adolescence the hormone surges stimulate the sebaceous glands to produce more sebum (oil).

WHAT DOES IT LOOK LIKE ON THE SKIN?

The excess sebum can lead to a risk of seborrhoea (excessively oily skin), enlarged pores, spots, blackheads and acne. Acne is more common in teen males due to the higher levels of testosterone.

WHAT CAN YOU DO TO HELP IT?

If you are going through puberty, the best thing you can do is take care of yourself by getting into a regular skincare routine. As a carer, the best thing you can do for a young person going through hormonal changes is to take them seriously.

ADULTS: Do not, under any circumstances, negate or dismiss a teenager's feelings if their skin is having a detrimental effect on their mental health. Take it, and them, seriously.

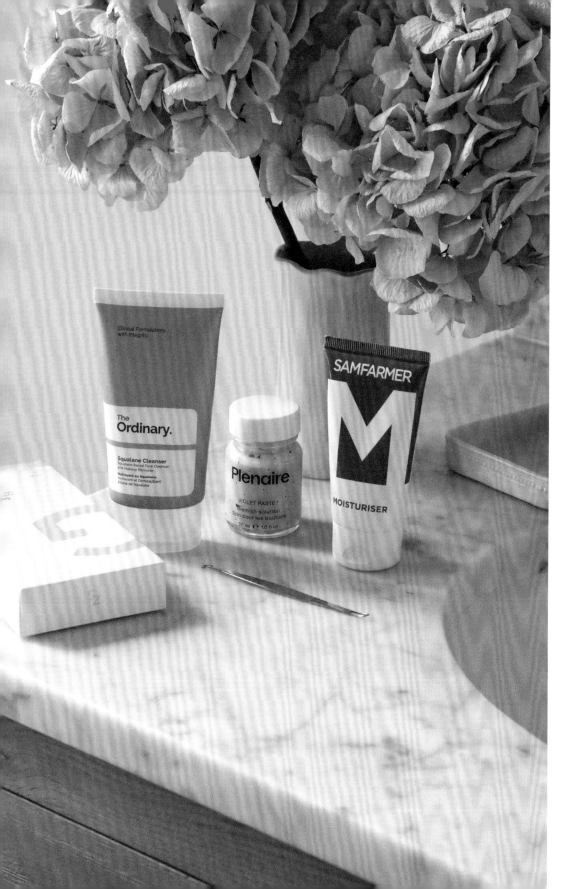

IF YOU ARE BUYING PRODUCTS FOR YOURSELF:

- Buy gentle products and use them regularly. Getting into a routine is the hardest part.
- Change pillowcases regularly (at least once a week), as they harbour bacteria.
- Use light oil-free moisturisers.
- Use spot treatments containing salicylic acid.
- Go for a professional treatment to encourage a good skincare routine and to pick the right products for your skin, remembering that not all teenage skins get spots.
- LED light is non-invasive and great for acneic younger skins.
- Fractional is more expensive, but it works.
- Do not be afraid to seek medical advice (or seek it on a teenager's behalf). That is what doctors are for.

WHAT SHOULD YOU AVOID?

- Avoid using harsh, drying 'traditional' acne products that strip the skin and leave it feeling tight and uncomfortable.
- Try not to relentlessly pick at spots.
- Wash your face regularly and keep it clean.
- I know from talking to a lot of clients that it can be tempting to wear a lot of makeup to cover your skin. Please make sure you are:

a) washing your brushes and sponges regularly
b) removing it all properly in the evening.

These two steps are imperative.

TRY THESE...

- Balance Me
- CeraVe
- La Roche-Posay
- Murad Clarifying Body Spray

- Murad Clarifying Oil-Free Water Gel
- Pestle & Mortar Superstar Retinoid Night Oil

- Plenaire (various)
- Sam Farmer – the entire range is for teens!
- ZitSticka (various)

PREGNANCY

WHAT HAPPENS?

Surges in hormones once again can cause all manner of upset in your skin.

WHAT DOES IT LOOK LIKE ON THE SKIN?

Pregnancy can make skin redder, puffier and give you breakouts that you may not have had before. It's not all bad, it can also give you a lovely, healthy, glow!

WHAT CAN YOU DO TO HELP IT?

- Invest in a hyaluronic facial mist to spray on your face when you are hot and flustered, or dry and dehydrated (or both). You'll also love it when you're in labour.
- Buy a quality fragrance-free facial oil if your skin is red and inflamed.
- Temporarily switch out your vitamin A/stronger skincare products, unless your doctor has told you to keep using them.
- Surges in hormones frequently result in breakouts, and despite old wives' tales, low levels of salicylic acid are completely safe for pregnant women. Doctors recommend using no higher than a 2 per cent product to tackle pregnancy breakouts, and most OTC products are sold at levels lower than 2 per cent.

WHAT SHOULD YOU AVOID?

- I would steer clear of using anything that your skin is not accustomed to during this period. Antagonising your skin it is risky because if you do find yourself with dermatitis, for example, you're limited in what you can do to treat it.
- Avoid strong retinoids (vitamin A), but do not panic if you see vitamin A listed lower down on the ingredients list of products that you use regularly. It is frequently used at low doses in skincare as part of the formula and is perfectly safe. When talking about retinoids in pregnancy, we are specifically referring to anything that stipulates vitamin A/retinol etc on the front of the pack.

TRY THESE...

- Clarins Tonic Treatment Oil (for stretch mark prevention)
- de Mamiel Pregnancy Facial Oil
- Medik8 Bakuchiol Peptides

PERIMENOPAUSE

WHAT HAPPENS?

Perimenopause and menopause cause the biggest changes to the skin. Oestrogen levels start to decrease in the skin up to 10 years before you turn fully menopausal. This has a knock-on effect with ceramides, the 'protective coat' around the epidermal skin cells, disrupting the skin barrier and making it harder for your skin to retain moisture. In the early stages of perimenopause, there is also more likely to be an imbalance between oestrogen and testosterone levels, which can lead to excessive hair, redness and spots.

WHAT DOES IT LOOK LIKE ON THE SKIN?

There is no one-size-fits-all to your skin's reaction to perimenopause. It depends on your hormones and obviously nothing is more individual. You may develop adult acne, rosacea, broken capillaries, dry skin, dull skin, rough skin. Or you may sail through with no changes in your skin at all. Lucky you! There is no way of predicting the effects of these massive hormonal fluctuations on your skin.

WHAT CAN YOU DO TO HELP IT?

As well as treating your skin as a 'maturing' one (see page 227), be aware of the following:
- You must keep an eye on your moles, as pre-cancer and cancerous changes become more common. Check your skin (and your boobs) more regularly.
- You will be more prone to bruising due to falling levels of oestrogen. Your skin literally becomes thinner.
- Your skin will be noticeably slower to heal. If you have an open wound that is not healing, and you suspect infection, seek medical help.

WHAT SHOULD YOU AVOID?

- Avoid jumping in with the latest 'miracle' ingredients claiming to 'replace lost collagen' in your skin. Those creams don't exist without a prescription. Save your money.
- If you do develop some breakouts, don't treat your skin as if you suddenly have full-blown acne. Your skin barrier is already compromised, and treating it aggressively will just add fuel to the fire. Treat the area, not the entire face.

MENOPAUSE (ah my people!)

WHAT HAPPENS?

The signs of ageing are accelerated and exaggerated, while the skin's ability to regenerate slows right down. Oestrogen is depleted, which has a huge knock-on effect on your body, your entire system and your skin. Consequently, ceramide, collagen and hyaluronic acid levels drop dramatically, and your skin is slower to heal. Your skin barrier is not as fortified as it needs to be.

WHAT DOES IT LOOK LIKE ON THE SKIN?

- This massive depletion of hormones leads to your skin losing tone, elasticity and its ability to retain moisture.
- The skin's built-in moisturising system needs oestrogen to work properly, so the absence of it can lead to dry, rough, flaky or itchy skin.
- Oestrogen is also responsible for high levels of sebum and hyaluronic acid in the skin so when it starts to deplete, you will find that it's even harder to retain moisture levels.
- Losing moisture means that your skin doesn't exfoliate itself properly, or in a speedy fashion. The enzymes that we need to allow exfoliation to happen are not optimised in dry skin, causing a build-up of skin cells. This leads to the aforementioned flakiness and even scales on the skin.
- Collagen fibres decrease in number, stiffen and break apart, resulting in deepened lines.
- Elastic fibres decrease and literally become looser. The fibres thicken and form clumps under the skin, resulting in visible wrinkles.

In short: menopausal skin can sometimes look dull, flat, sagging (sorry), dry, wrinkled and like it's lost its glow.

WHAT CAN YOU DO TO HELP IT?

Worry ye not. Help is at hand. There are a multitude of things that you can do to offset any signs of ageing that you do not want to see on your face. As there is no way of knowing which way your skin will react in menopause, especially early menopause when your hormones are still capable of fluctuating wildly, I've divided my advice by skin condition:

Dry/dull/lost its 'oomph'

CLEANSERS: milks and creams work well on an older skin. They don't aggravate the barrier when you're trying to remove it like a heavy-duty cleansing balm can sometimes do, and they are gentle enough to cause no further harm. If your skin is redder than usual during this period, it may be worth avoiding fragranced products.

SERUMS: this depends on what your skin can handle. On the one hand, there is an argument for upping the ante with things like retinoids/vitamin A, and on the other, there is not exactly a lot of 'collagen' waiting around in your skin for your products to 'stimulate', a claim the industry tends to frequently throw around with abandon.

Listen to your skin. If you are experiencing redness, sensitivity and the odd red, sore breakout that won't heal, try limiting your skincare to cleansing, maybe misting (for light hydration and for the cooling effect), moisturising and SPF for daytime. Repeat, minus the SPF, for the evening. Look for products that use terms such as 'barrier repair' and that contain ingredients such as ceramides and amino acids.

MOISTURISERS: we as an industry tend to push older women to thicker, richer, more emollient creams, and this is not always what they need. We've come a long way since the days of Helena Rubinstein's Valaze and Estée Lauder's initial foray into richer, luxurious moisturisers like Super Rich All-Purpose Cream.

If your skin feels as dry as a desert, even itchy, try a thicker cream than you might have used in your 20s and 30s. If it feels like it needs a little more 'juice', use lighter moisturisers that have a higher water content as opposed to oil. These are easy to spot and test in store. They feel lighter on your skin and penetrate very quickly.

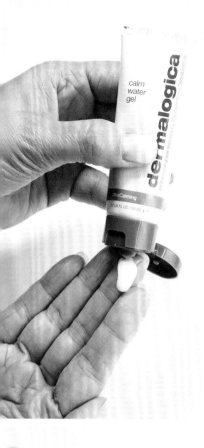

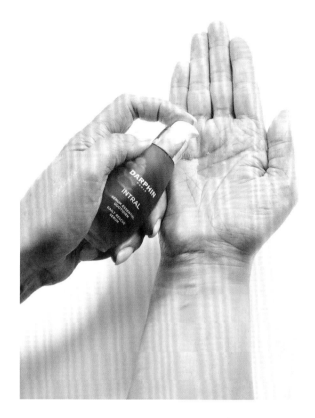

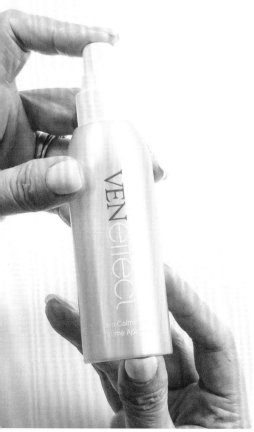

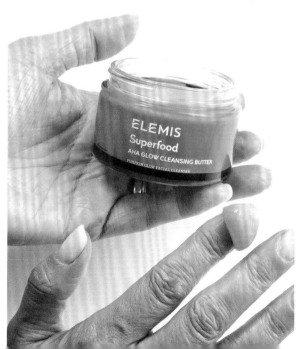

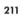

Onset of adult acne/lots of breakouts/oily skin

CLEANSERS: light gels, milks and creams for this skin type are fine. The newer foaming cleansers are also good but stay away from the traditional foaming products that can leave your skin uncomfortable, tight and sore.

Newer foams tend to exclude SLS (sodium lauryl sulphate) and use more gentle derivatives such as coconut for their foaming element. They may also have a mechanical foaming action, so look liquid in the packaging then pump out into a soft foam. These are generally light and easy on the skin.

SERUMS: if you are suffering with breakouts, look for serums or treatments containing either retinoids/vitamin A, niacinamide or azelaic acid. They work well on an older skin that is throwing its toys out of the pram.

MOISTURISERS: go for oil-free, lighter formulations that will hydrate your skin rather than placing further oil onto it. These products will nearly always be labelled 'oil-free' somewhere on the front of the pack, which will save you trying to read an ingredients label. If your skin is reddened and has breakouts, avoid fragranced products. They can exacerbate an angry barrier.

WHAT SHOULD YOU AVOID?

- Across all categories, avoid jumping in with aggressive ingredients, products or treatments. It can overwhelm the skin and cause further irritation. If you want to invest in a serum that is dedicated to your skin condition, do so, but make an informed decision. Don't buy on a whim, save your money.
- Avoid using strong acids, retinoids and other actives all together in one sitting, it's too much for an older skin.

PCOS AND ENDOMETRIOSIS

WHAT HAPPENS?

Polycystic Ovary Syndrome (PCOS) is a hormone disorder in women of reproductive age that causes a large number of underdeveloped sacs (follicles) in your ovary to struggle to produce an egg each month or to swell with excess fluid.

Endometriosis is a medical condition where cells similar to those lining the womb are found elsewhere in the body. They react in the same way as those lining the womb and break down each month and cause a bleed. The problem being, of course, that where the womb would shed its lining and you would have a period, there is no escape for the blood in the cells outside of the womb.

WHAT DOES IT LOOK LIKE ON THE SKIN?

I paired these conditions together because they can have a similar effect on your skin and are treated, skincare-wise, in much the same way.

- PCOS can present with acne, which usually shows on the lower part of the face, including the jawline, chin and upper neck. People with PCOS may find that their acne is deeper, larger and takes longer to heal.
- Hirsutism, or excessive hair growth in places where hair is usually absent or minimal, is also a sign of PCOS that shows on the skin. Most commonly found on the chin, neck, abdomen, chest and back.
- Balding or thinning of the hair can be seen on the scalp – and both of these hair issues are driven by an excess of testosterone.
- A big concern for sufferers of endometriosis is the inconsistency of their skin. It can look fine one day and the next be hit with any of the following:
  - **Hives**: people with endo tend to be more allergy-prone, frequently resulting in reactions on their skin to common irritants, and random, unexpected ones.
  - **Dermatitis** is more common with endometriosis.
  - **Acne**: as with PCOS, endometriosis can cause acne on the lower half of the face, usually around the time of a period.
  - **Eczema and psoriasis**: higher levels of inflammation in the body are thought to contribute to the higher rates of these skin conditions in people with endometriosis.

WHAT CAN YOU DO TO HELP IT?

The effects of PCOS and endometriosis on the skin are best treated by causing no further harm.

- If you present with acne, follow the recommendations for that condition on pages 82–87.
- Aim for fragrance-free products that use terms like 'soothing' and 'calming'.
- Invest in a calming mist or serum to help your skin when it's flaring.
- Find a nicely hydrating moisturiser that isn't too heavy on the skin. The main ingredient listed first on the ingredient list should be water, not oil.

WHAT SHOULD YOU AVOID?

- Try to avoid known skin irritants such as rough scrubs, fragrance (synthetic and natural), and strong ingredients such as camphor, eucalyptus, mint and menthol.
- No harsh abrasives such as scrubs or mechanical cleansing brushes.
- Stay away from high levels of alcohol in your skincare products.
- If your skin is red, irritated and suffering, avoid strong active ingredients in your routine, such as retinoids, some more intense acids and some vitamin C products.

TRY THESE...

My recommendations for Perimenopause, Menopause, PCOS and Endometriosis are very similar, as they are based on fluctuating hormones and what they can do to your skin. As ever, use what works for you.

- Darphin Intral range
- Dermalogica Calm Water Gel and UltraCalming™ range
- Dr. Andrew Weil for Origins™ Mega-Mushroom range
- Dr.Jart+™ Ceramidin and Cicapair™ ranges
- Elemis Superfood AHA Glow Cleansing Butter

- La Roche-Posay Toleriane Ultra 8 Mist
- REN Evercalm™ range
- The Ordinary Natural Moisturizing Factors +HA
- The Ordinary Squalane Cleanser
- VENeffect Skin Calming Mist
- Votary Super Seed range (fragrance free but does include essential oils)

" LISTEN TO YOUR SKIN "

CHRONIC ILLNESS

If you have an auto-immune disease that causes skin inflammation and flare-ups, such as multiple sclerosis, lupus or perhaps even depression or ME:

- If you are having a flare-up, avoid stimulating ingredients such as acids and exfoliators. They can be too abrasive on a skin that is already stressed.
- Use soothing cleansers, facial oils and moisturisers. You may be able to use slightly more active products if you are not in the middle of a flare-up/episode, but you know your body and skin better than anyone else.
- Consider using fragrance-free products if you think fragrance is aggravating your skin. If you have broken skin as a result of your illness, fragrance may well irritate your barrier further.

However, some people find that the ritual of their self-care routine is vital to their well-being and is enhanced with fragranced products. Do what feels good to you, both physically and mentally.

CHEMOTHERAPY

Chemo has a strong impact on your skin and will require changes to your usual routine. The job of chemotherapy is to kill your cancerous cells and prevent them from reproducing and growing. Unfortunately, it also has this effect on healthy cells, leading to very dry and fragile, and more sensitive, skin.

At a time when your immune system is already compromised, a damaged skin barrier can leave you even more prone to infection. Your skin barrier needs to be fortified and strengthened as much as possible in order to cope with chemotherapy's side effects.

Everything in your kit should be geared towards protecting your skin from the outside in. Think of it as fully closing a door that has been left slightly ajar. Chemotherapy can leave the skin red, sore, irritated, itchy, blistered and extremely dry. This is a time for treating your skin delicately, and with the goal to nourish and protect, not stimulate.

- Cut out most of your active products, including anything like scrubs, acids and retinoids. Exfoliation is not required during this period.

- Avoid using alcohol, fragrance and essential oils directly on the skin. They can all be especially irritating on a disrupted skin barrier.

- Try to switch to a zinc oxide-based physical sunscreen and use SPF30+. Some chemotherapy drugs may also cause a sun allergy, so ensure that you are taking your doctor's advice and covering up well.

- Chemotherapy drugs can cause severe disruption to the nail bed. This can, again, leave you extremely susceptible to infection, so keep nails short and do not, however tempting it is, pick at your nails or cuticles.

- Avoid taking hot showers and baths. Ensure the water is warm, not hot.

- Try not to scratch or rub your skin. Wear loose clothing to prevent skin irritation and heat on the surface of your skin.

- Your skin will continue to be sensitised and vulnerable for a certain period after your last treatment finishes. Talk to your doctor before reintroducing your normal products to your routine. It is also common to be left extremely sun-sensitive for an extended period after treatment. Bear this in mind, go easy and always listen to your doctor's advice.

TRY THESE...

Some people going through chemotherapy have told me they've found the following helpful, but always check your product choices with your oncologist first.

- Biossance 100% Squalane Oil

- Dermalogica Barrier Defense Booster

- Dermalogica Ultracalming Barrier Repair

- Pai Rosehip BioRegenerate Oil

- Zelens Power D Treatment Drops

Try the product recommendations for sensitive skins on page 68

THE BARE MINIMUM

The joy of doing in-person events is that I get to talk to a lot of you in a much more intimate fashion than via the internet. It's not unusual for up to five people each day to share that they would normally have struggled to attend something quite so loud/busy/frenetic due to various conditions such as ME, fibromyalgia, depression, anxiety or other serious illnesses such as MS.

Honestly, the only reason I advocate attempting any kind of skin 'care' in all of these situations is purely for the self-care aspect.

On days where you think 'I can't face moving' – for whatever reason – do the absolute bare minimum and don't give yourself a hard time about it.

When you can't face much, but want to do 'something', keep these skincare routine tips to hand: they're affordable, easy and not too active.

CLEANSING

Wipes. Yes – there is the odd wipe that isn't atrocious (in this situation):

Water wipes are literally water, with a natural preservative to keep them fresh. If I still had small people these would be my wipe of choice. They're enough to freshen you up if you can't move. In 'all' areas.

RMS Beauty Ultimate Makeup Remover Wipes only contain coconut oil and shouldn't do any further harm if you need something to feel a little more substantial for your face than the water wipes. You need to hold the packet in your hand for a few minutes to heat up the coconut oil and ensure it's melted in the sachet before you open it.

Don't flush any wipes down the toilet.

MOISTURISING

Moisturiser-wise there are plenty of good, nourishing options for affordable, soothing, calming products that get to work on your skin without causing irritation: you can literally stick them on your face and forget about them.

Just do what you can. When you can.

TRY THESE...

- **Squalane oil** is one of my first recommendations for anyone with a reactive, reddened, sensitised skin. It is a great light, moisturising facial oil for all skin types, and it's fragrance-free so won't irritate you if you are also sensitive to smell. A little goes a long way, so use it sparingly.

- **Serozinc** is a great refreshing mist/hydrator for all skins, not just the oily/combination skin types that it was traditionally marketed for. It's soft, sprays a lovely light mist and is suitable for misting at all times, not just after cleansing.

- **Weleda Skin Food** is still one of my favourites for a face that just wants comfort and/or moisturising. The newer, lighter version is much better for you if you have oily/combination skin. It's a must-have for most skins and most kits, to be honest. It needs warming gently with the fingers before application (an exception to my 'products don't need warming in the hands' rule – page 45).

- **REN Evercalm™ range** is designed with sensitive or stressed skin in mind, and contains a product for every stage of your routine.

- Zelens Youth Concentrate Supreme Age-Defying Serum.

- Kate Somerville +Retinol Vitamin C Moisturiser

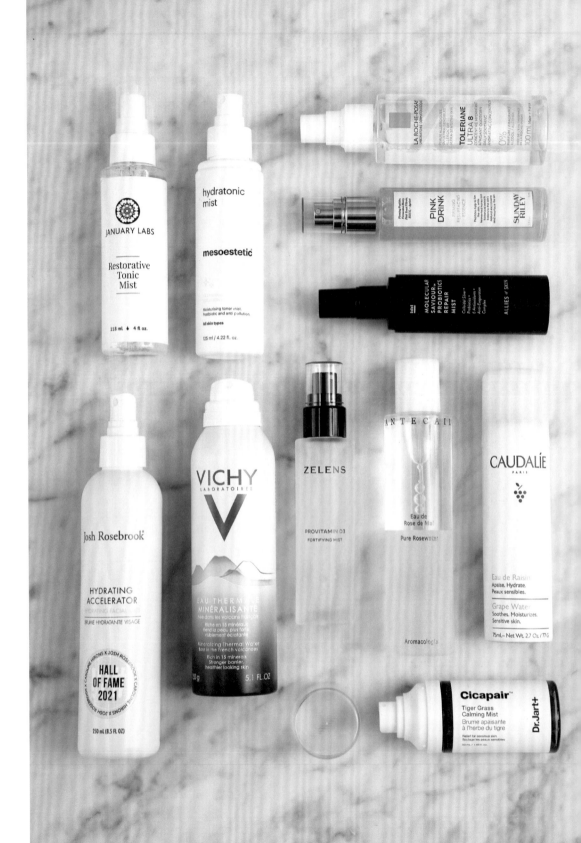

ROUTINE FOR DRY, DEHYDRATED OR PARCHED SKIN

Dehydrated skin can seem like it would need a whole new routine, but actually the foundations are exactly the same. These are the situations and products you'll want to focus on to help quench your skin's thirst.

#CLEANSER

Stay away from harsh, foaming cleansers. I know I say this all the time, but it's particularly important when your epidermis already resembles a prune. Stick to cleansing milks, oils or creams. They will help plump up your skin and enable it to retain moisture from your very first step. Using an SLS-laden foaming cleanser on a dry, parched, dehydrated skin is akin to skin torture and is a skincare crime of the highest order. Please bear that in mind whenever you see the term 'recommended by dermatologists' or 'approved by dermatologists'. Derms don't do that for free. Someone is getting paid.

#ACIDS

Keep using acids, but consider switching to lactic acid, which is good for surface exfoliation.

#MISTS OR SPRITZ

This is key and your best friend. You'll be using these liberally until your skin feels better. Layer moisture between every step in your skincare routine to give the feeling that your skin is hydrated. 'Mist' or 'spritz' always means using a spray that contains hyaluronic acid, which locks in moisture, not just plain water in a spray bottle or tin.

▌ Fake it 'til you make it.

#SERUMS/OILS

Apply a hyaluronic-based serum to your skin, let it soak in, spritz, and spritz again if necessary. If this isn't enough, you can apply an oil on top. I tend to use oil-based serums or full facial oils when my skin feels really dry and dehydrated.

With this skin situation, silicone-based serums tend to 'roll' more and don't feel like they are doing their job. Wait a week or so before introducing them. The easiest way to tell if your product is silicone-based without the aid of the ingredient list is to apply half a pump to the back of your hand. If it is absorbed immediately, it's silicone; if there is residue on the skin and the product seems to spread all over your hand, it's probably oil-heavy.

#SPRITZ AGAIN

I cannot say this enough. YOU CAN NEVER SPRITZ TOO MUCH.

#MOISTURISER

This is not a time to go oil-free. You need oil in your moisturiser to help lock in the moisture.

Think of the top layers of the skin as a sponge that is emerging halfway out of a bowl of water. The top part of the skin is drying out and exposed. A common mistake when treating dry, dehydrated or parched skin is to apply a thick layer of moisturiser. This is akin to applying a thick layer of cold butter to cold toast. It won't penetrate – it will sit on the surface of the skin and/or roll off. Don't waste your product. Apply just enough moisturiser on top of your oil or serum to give comfort to your skin. Wait a little while, *spritz again*, then reapply a little moisturiser. In scientific terms you would normally apply oil last, as the molecules are bigger than those in moisturisers. However, for ease of wearing makeup and a non-sticky feeling on the face, I like to apply my moisturiser last. And in this case, it's nice to seal in the oil or serum. If you're not wearing makeup, you can repeat thin layers of moisturiser throughout the day. Cleanse as usual in the evening and do your normal routine. Repeat as before, until your skin feels more comfortable.

LIPS

Include your lips in your entire routine when they're dry. Just be gentle...

Cleanse them, use your acid pads over them, even if it's just around the edges – if they are split it will sting like hell, so go with your instinct (a word of warning: I have yet to taste a nice acid), use your oil on them, and use your moisturiser on them. Reapply a little oil as needed throughout the day. They will improve quickly with a little TLC.

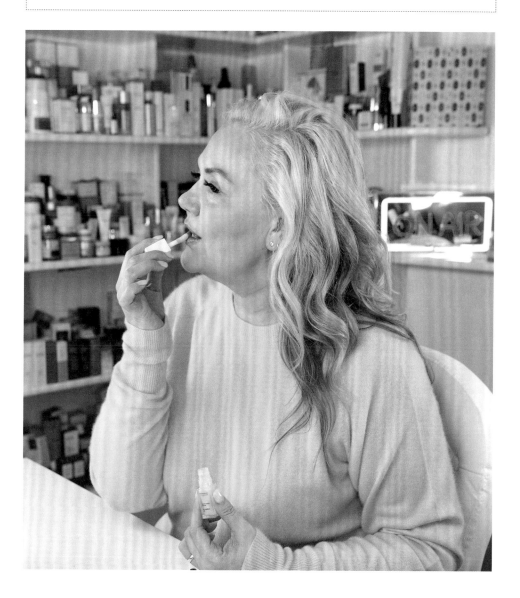

CELLULITE CREAMS WORK

FACT: Cellulite is not caused by trapped 'toxins'. If we were as 'toxic' as some parts of the 'wellness' industry would have us believe, we'd all be dead. A long time ago.

FACT: Cellulite is caused when your underlying fat cells start to push through connective tissue. Connective tissue is weakened by a mixture of things, including hormones, lack of exercise, poor muscle tone, excess fat and poor circulation.

FACT: 90 per cent of women get cellulite, compared to 10 per cent of men. Men have stronger connective tissue. They still have fat underneath it, it's just not as easy for it to escape. How rude.

FACT: It gets worse for women as we age. Lack of oestrogen makes it worse.

FACT: It's in your genes. Look at your mum and grandmother. If they have it...

FACT: Some fillers and injectables can help – albeit temporarily – but they only really work on very slim people who have the odd 'dent' rather than full-blown cellulite legs. Think models before catwalk shows/big shoots.

FACT: Lasers, massage (specific for this problem) and radio-frequency treatments can help, but again it will only be temporary. And it takes a ton of sessions. Personally, I think your time would be better spent at the gym/ walking for an hour, rather than lying flat out letting someone pound the area in vain...

FACT: Liposuction does nothing. It's like removing a bit of stuffing from a pillow. It leaves an indentation and doesn't magically spread the fat around nice and neatly.

FACT: Water helps. Eating veg that are water-heavy and drinking a lot of water throughout the day, every day, helps. It doesn't fix it, but it can help.

FACT: Smoking makes cellulite worse, as it weakens connective tissue (collagen). See opposite page.

FACT: There is not one cellulite cream on the market that gets rid of cellulite. Not one. Either by prescription or over the counter, it makes no difference. They may make your skin feel softer and smoother, but they aren't shifting the fat.

Eat well, move around more, drink plenty of water, take care of your health in general. And even after you've done all that, your genes may well just insist that you keep your cellulite.

Save your money.

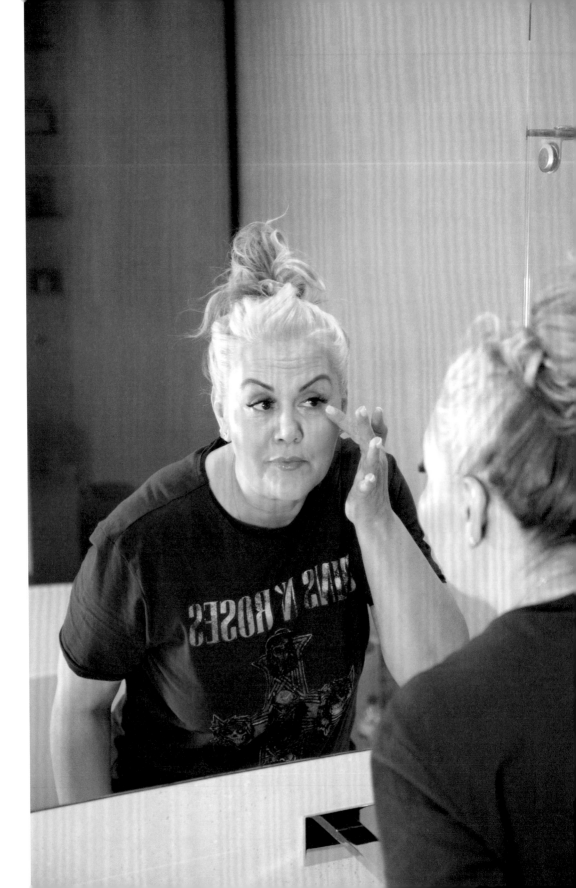

WHEN SHOULD I START USING ANTI-AGEING PRODUCTS?

SPF: technically from birth, but most companies won't advocate using SPF until your baby is 6 months old. Keep them protected from direct sunlight.

VITAMIN A: if you have acne you may be prescribed a retinoid by your doctor. Otherwise, around 30+, depending on lifestyle – if you're a sun worshipper and/or you smoke, you can start earlier.

GLYCOLIC/LACTIC/SALICYLIC ACIDS: again, this depends on lifestyle and skin type. If you have acne you can use salicylic acid topically. The other two can be introduced from the age of 25+ as needed.

VITAMINS C AND E: from the word go. As soon as you start your skincare routine choose something with these in. Good move.

NIACINAMIDE: 25+ ish, again depending on lifestyle and skin type. Acne? Crack on.

The basic thing to remember is that, for women, our collagen production is linked directly to our ovaries. When we are at our most fertile our skin is usually at its best. As you near menopause and go through perimenopause you will notice huge changes in your entire system, not just your skin. Hitting menopause has a direct link to your collagen. It's a bit like someone takes away a little of the scaffolding that supports your facial structure with each passing year.

So, start taking care of your skin when you get your periods, and step it up a notch when you get to 35+ (especially if you go into early menopause or have a full hysterectomy).

And when you do start using these products, do not forget your SPF.

And if you smoke? Scrap all that advice and use all of the above – now.

'ANTI-AGEING' PRODUCTS

'Anti-ageing'. We're all so used to this term that we don't even question it. If a product says it is 'anti-ageing' on the box, then it must be, right?

Wrong.

Remember, old is the goal. I don't like the term anti-ageing – if we're lucky enough, we all get older – but the industry is slow to catch up and still thinks youth is the dream. So, until we come up with a better solution, this is what we're stuck with.

If ever a phrase has been over-used, anti-ageing is the one. Few ingredients are indeed 'anti-ageing', but some are entitled to be called 'ageing prevention' as they do not reverse signs of ageing, but they do help slow them down or prevent them from getting worse.

The next time you pick up a product that claims to be anti-ageing, what you need to look out for is one of these:

SPF

SPF is anti-ageing. It has been proven, undoubtedly, unequivocally. Although if you're younger you could argue that it belongs in the 'prevention' category. It doesn't fix damage that has already been done. That is the job of...

VITAMIN A

Vitamin A is the only other ingredient, along with SPF, that the FDA will legally let manufacturers claim to be anti-ageing in the USA. Vitamin A reverses the signs of ageing. It rebuilds collagen, repairs sun damage and is an all-round good egg. There are various derivatives of vitamin A – if you have previously used a product with vitamin A in it and reacted badly, it may just be that you haven't yet found the right one for you (see pages 130–135).

GLYCOLIC/LACTIC/SALICYLIC ACIDS

Acids used in the right way can be beneficial to the skin. When applied as topical exfoliants they resurface the epidermis, allowing better product penetration and, in the case of some well-formulated AHAs, help rebuild collagen. Glycolic and lactic acids are better for a drier skin, and salicylic acid is better for oily/combination skin. Don't opt for a very strong product straight away, and do not go mad. Less is sometimes more.

VITAMINS C AND E

These two work well together, as vitamin C is traditionally water-based (newer formulas include oil-based vitamin C) and vitamin E is oil-based, thus protecting both the oil and water parts of the cell. Both are antioxidants, so sit in the 'prevention' category.

NIACINAMIDE

This is vitamin B3 by another name. When used on the skin it has been shown to stimulate the dermis and in turn increase the fatty content of the cells, along with helping the skin retain water. As it is shown to enhance the barrier function of the epidermis (thereby protecting the skin against bacterial attack) it has had good results with acne sufferers.

Other ingredients are beneficial to the skin in other ways, but if anti-ageing is the aim you need some of these in your product (not all of them at once). See page 227 on when you should start using them.

TRY THESE...

- Alpha-H Vitamin Profiling Kit

- Kate Somerville Retinol Vitamin C + Moisturiser

- Medik8 Vitamin A and C range

- Paula's Choice 10% Niacinamide Booster

- The Ordinary Niacinamide 10% + Zinc 1%

- Zelens Youth Concentrate

SPOTS

Zits. Pustules. Papules. Wheals. Comedones. Milia. There are lots of things that happen to the skin – especially on the face – on a regular basis.

This is purely about SPOTS.

Acne? I'm not talking to you. Blackheads? Nor you. Pustules? Nope. I'm talking about your average spot that pops up occasionally. You know it's coming – you can feel it. It starts with a bump, feels sore, then gets a little red, hurts a little more, then you see a faint hint of something that could be a head. A little white may show underneath.

And then, typically, if you are the average person, you:

- Stab it (leading to scarring)
- Poke it (does absolutely nothing)
- Squeeze it (if you do this too early, the skin will bruise, then potentially scar)
- Load it with tea tree oil (no need – it's probably not bacterial)
- Load it with spot treatment (see above)
- or GOD FORBID – put toothpaste on it (please, no)

Toothpaste. Paste for TEETH. On a spot. **No.**

Next time you feel one of these mothers coming up you will need the following:

- Your hands
- Your moisturiser/a good facial oil
- Your concealer
- Patience

Moisturise the area like it's going out of fashion.

Yes, really. This is particularly good for those big on-the-chin, once-a-month spots. Moisturising it does a few things: it softens the area around the spot – how often have you destroyed the surrounding area of a zit because you treated the area of the said zit so abusively? – and then either makes the spot retreat entirely OR brings it to a head quicker – in which case you have my permission to pop. Pop pop away (see pages 232–235).

WORDS OF WARNING

A 'popable' spot shouldn't really hurt when popping – it should be satisfying.

If it hurts – stop – it's too soon and you will bruise and then possibly scar.

Stop at the first sign of blood – you're about to scar.

Never, ever, ever try to pop milia (see pages 96–99). Get them removed professionally.

The next time you feel Mount Vesuvius brewing under the skin give it a chance, treat it with care and save the toothpaste for your mouth. Please.

HOW TO
POP A SPOT

As much as any dermatologist will tell you not to pop, the fact is that you do.
We do. You know you do; I know you do; the industry at large knows that you
do, but they pretend that you don't. I know there are some of you that manage to
restrain yourselves, but you're in the minority and up there with those people that
don't lick their lips when eating a doughnut or chew when eating a fruit pastille.
You exist, but the rest of us don't know how you manage it.

I'm a popper. Always have been.
There's nothing more satisfying to be honest.

And I know most of you pop because you tell me so – usually with 'don't shout
at me' eyes. As if! If it's the right time, I always pop. With that in mind, I offer
you *my* way to pop. All risk is your own.

Please bear in mind: **Popping is not picking.** They are two very different things.

How so?

Popping – 'Ooh I see a whitehead! Where did that come from? I think I can get that out. Let me have a go. Yep. Excellent.' *carries on with routine*

Picking – 'Ow. That red lump on my chin is KILLING ME. I must be due on. Bloody hormones. I'm going to get it out.' *attempts to pop red lump for ages*
'OWWW. Ugh. I'll try again later. Ooh there's another one! Maybe that one will come out.' *prods second bump until it bleeds*
'OOWWWW. Ugh. No joy. Why does my skin hate me?'
plays with it all day with dirty fingers, doesn't leave it alone

If you fall into the latter category, you're making the simple mistake of opening the oven door before the cake has risen. A little patience changes the outcome.

A few simple guidelines will give the best result (although do bear in mind that every skin is different) and they will probably go against everything you've read from brands trying to sell you products. Nothing new there, so let's crack on.

WHAT YOU WILL NEED:

'Clean' everything. Clean hands. Clean skin. Clean flannel. Clean tissue. Acids. Cotton pads or a ready-made acid pad. A good-quality (non-mineral oil) facial oil.

- Slipping it into your routine is the easiest way. AM or PM. Not lunchtime in the loo at work.

- Cleanse. With a clean flannel. If the flannel doesn't knock the head off the spot that's your first sign that it may not be ready. If it's sore, it's probably not ready. I steer clear of sore spots. They're still working their way up the dermis food chain and causing inflammation along the way. Soak a cotton pad with acid toner and set it aside (or unpack your ready-made acid pad).

- If you can see white, it's not sore or too tender and everything is clean, take a tissue, rip it in half and wrap it around the forefinger of each hand.

- Finger placement is also crucial. One of the biggest mistakes made when popping is to go straight in from RIGHT NEXT TO THE SPOT. You put your two fingers on the spot and you just push your fingers together, so that you're so close, you literally just get a little teeny whitehead, then everything almost gets pushed back down into the spot. Not good.

- Do NOT use your nails. Use the pads of your fingertips only.

- Put your fingers either side of the spot, as best you can, depending on where it is, obviously. You should be able to SEE the spot. Gently push downwards and then, at a 90-degree angle towards the bottom the spot, start to push upwards. If it's ready, it will come up and out. Gently repeat. When the white stops, and it's spouting pink, STOP. STOP. STOP. STOP.

- If you see blood (it's already too late but...), STOP. You're in scarring territory. Show restraint.

- Now you need to move quickly. Take your pre-soaked acid toner cotton pad, or ready-and-waiting acid pad and apply it firmly to the spot, using a similar pressure as when you've ripped off a plaster or a wax strip. Hard pressure. Hold it down for a few seconds, then turn it over and repeat. There should be no bleeding. If there is, keep the acid on it until it stops. I have been known to walk around making a cup of tea while holding an acid-soaked pad on an overly pronged spot waiting for it to calm itself. The bigger the spot, the longer you hold acid on it.

  Note: this may sting like a MOFO (technical term). Stinging is good. I know I say it all the time, but stinging is good. The acid will be helping to kill the bacteria, helping it heal quicker and making sure the skin is prepped ready for the oil. You'll have a 'Kevin at the sink in *Home Alone*' moment. Embrace it.

- Yes, oil. I don't use drying-out products. If you dry out the spot, you also dry out the area surrounding the spot, causing a ton of inflammation and dehydration and, frankly, making a prime breeding ground for bacteria and scarring. A Juicy Lucy skin is harder to scar. A dried-out, shrivelled-up area will scar easily. Simples.

- Take your acid pad off and put your chosen oil on the area.

- Massage it firmly in. You can't be namby-pamby at this stage. Be firm. Use good, strong pressure, massaging all around the spot and over the spot.

- Depending on the rest of your day/evening, finish your routine, but I try to do this either on mornings that I'm not wearing makeup and am working from home, or in the evenings at teatime.

- It's best to do it when you're at home with a little time afterwards as you're going to repeat the oil application as soon as it has all been absorbed... Apply, wait, absorb, apply, wait, absorb. Repeat at least three times if you can.

- Throughout the day or the next morning, you will find that the spot erupts a little goo, like a mini volcano. Wipe this away with acid and reapply the oil. This sounds time-consuming but I promise we're talking seconds, not hours. And it's worth it if it speeds up the spot healing process and helps prevent scarring.

- If you have a ready spot but you have to go to work, do everything as above, apply your moisturiser over the area, don't avoid it – and then proceed with your makeup. Powder is your friend. Once you get home, cleanse immediately and do it all again. You may find the rest of the spot just throws itself at you willingly, or that it has calmed significantly to be almost invisible. Just don't be tempted to start on it like you're climbing Everest with a pickaxe.

The reason I use oil on spots, rather than drying products, is because in my experience, drying them out doesn't always work and causes more damage. Using oil does one of two things: it either swells up the spot and forces the 'head' of the spot to show up the next morning, or it settles it down and almost disperses the remnants.

There are, of course, 'extraction tools' available on the market, but you can't use them where you can't see the spot, and you need to know how much pressure is too much.

Freckles are cute. At any age.
You will do damage to your skin trying
to get rid of them. Leave them alone.
Embrace them.

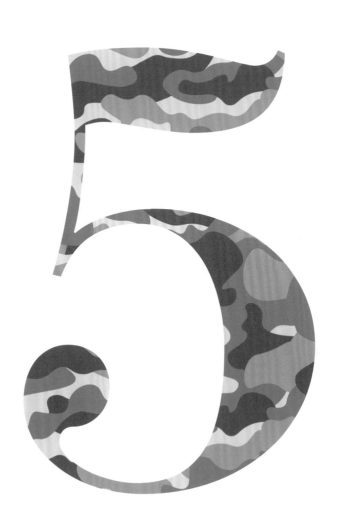

THINK SCIENCE

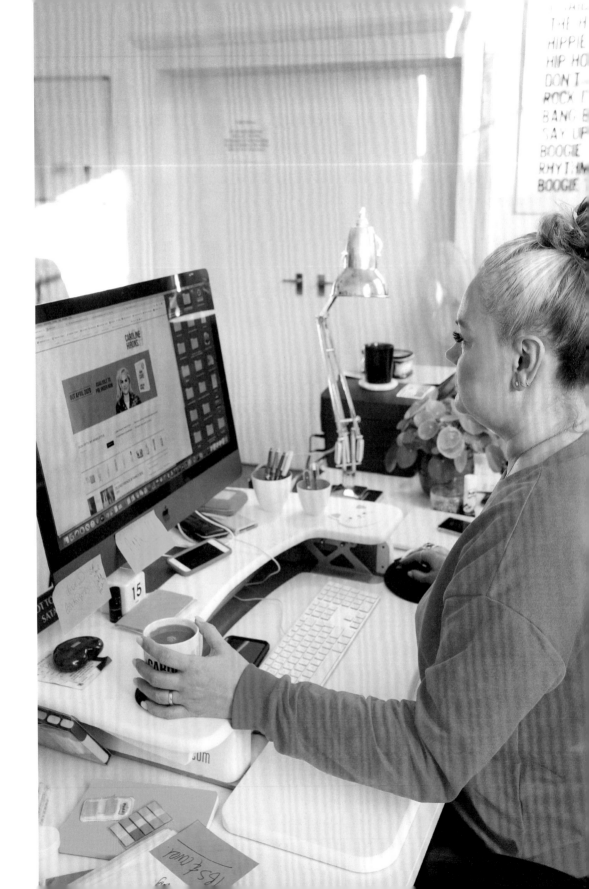

WELCOME TO THE INDUSTRY!

So, by now you should have a better idea what your skin type is, how to treat it, and the products you need. Well, here's the thing. The skincare industry makes a lot of money by confusing you. The more knowledge you have about the products available, the less likely you are to be persuaded to purchase something that you do not need. Whether you're reading packaging or are getting assaulted by social media ads, the terminology is a minefield. So let's break it down Jilly Cooper style and meet the heroes and villains in the world of skincare – the industry jargon – and bust those overused, misused, confusing and downright pointless words and phrases. I want the skincare industry to be taken seriously, and what better way to start than with a healthy dose of reality.

HYPO-ALLERGENIC

Literally means 'should not cause an allergy', which to be honest is a fairly meaningless term. There's no industry or legal standard to back this up, and there are different standards worldwide. Ultimately, this is just **lip service**. What is an extreme allergen to you may be perfectly fine for me.

IS ABSORBED IMMEDIATELY

You will find this claim on products that contain synthetic pushers. These force the product into the skin. Most serums that aren't completely natural or organic contain synthetic pushers. Your skin is highly intelligent – it's not going to absorb anything in a hurry in case it's harmful to you. If it did, we wouldn't need patches for things like HRT and injections for insulin. Its job is to be a barrier. If a product is absorbed straight away, it's not natural (which is fine). (See page 240 for more on what 'natural' means.)

ANIMAL TESTING

Poor animal lovers. Talk about a minefield. Unless a brand categorically states 'against animal testing' or 'no animal testing' on its product, assume it may sell in territories that require animal testing. Just because a brand doesn't test its *final* product on animals, doesn't mean that all of the ingredients weren't tested on animals in the past. But this is inevitable, and not something that should make you question the brand's ethics. Animal testing is banned in the EU and Australia, but sticklers will point to certain territories internationally and say they won't support a brand because the product is sold there. That is obviously your call, but the fact remains that nothing you put on your face in the UK was tested on an animal in order for you to use it. It is also worth noting that many of these territories have a cross-border policy that makes it possible to sell a product in that country without it being tested on animals.

If you want to know categorically where a brand stands, you need to ask them: 'Are your ingredients tested on animals *at their source?*' and 'Do you retail in territories where the government requires animal testing?' If they don't know, assume they are.

A brand that cares about animal testing will ensure its standards are met from the very beginning of the production process and will shout it from the rooftops.

NATURAL

The most over-used and abused word in the industry.

> I could take a cup of glue, a sip of aloe vera juice, spit the aloe vera juice into the glue, label it 'natural' and sell it as a skincare product.

There is no legal guideline or industry standard for the word 'natural'. It's all about marketing. If a product is labelled 'natural' you think you're doing yourself some good. Read the label. Educate yourself. There are, *of course*, excellent brands out there that would place themselves in the 'natural' category. There are also some heinous ones. And a word to the wise – the misinformation and scare-mongering is worse when it comes to baby products. Outrageous.

NON-COMEDOGENIC

This literally means 'does not block pores'. Where to start? All evidence that a product is 'non-comedogenic' is anecdotal. It is unproven and untested scientifically. Pure, naturally derived lanolin is supposed to be a 'non-comedogenic' alternative to synthetic lanolin, but if I put any kind of lanolin anywhere near my face it will be covered in huge whiteheads within hours. Use it as a rough guide rather than the word of law.

ORGANIC

This is marginally better than 'natural', as at least there are *some* standards in place, however, the Soil Association, Ecocert and all the numerous international organic certification bodies have different standards between them. You'd need to go directly to their websites to see if your standards match theirs. See page 282.

SHRINKS PORES

Pores are not doors – they do not open and close.

Nothing opens and closes pores. There is a big fat difference between saying 'closes pores' and 'minimises the appearance of pores'. One is rubbish and the other is a possibility.

SILKY SMOOTH

Contains silicone. Check the INCI list – anything ending in '...cone' or '...one' is a silicone. I actually don't mind silicones at all, but let's be clear *why* the product is silky smooth.

VELVETY SOFT

See above.

DERMATOLOGIST-TESTED

This has no legal standing or definition. It also does not mean that the product tested 'positively' by a derm, just that it was 'tested'. 'How was it tested?' you may ask? Probably by rubbing a bit on their hand, or on a patient's face, to check for any reaction. It is a genuinely pointless term and I pay no attention to it.

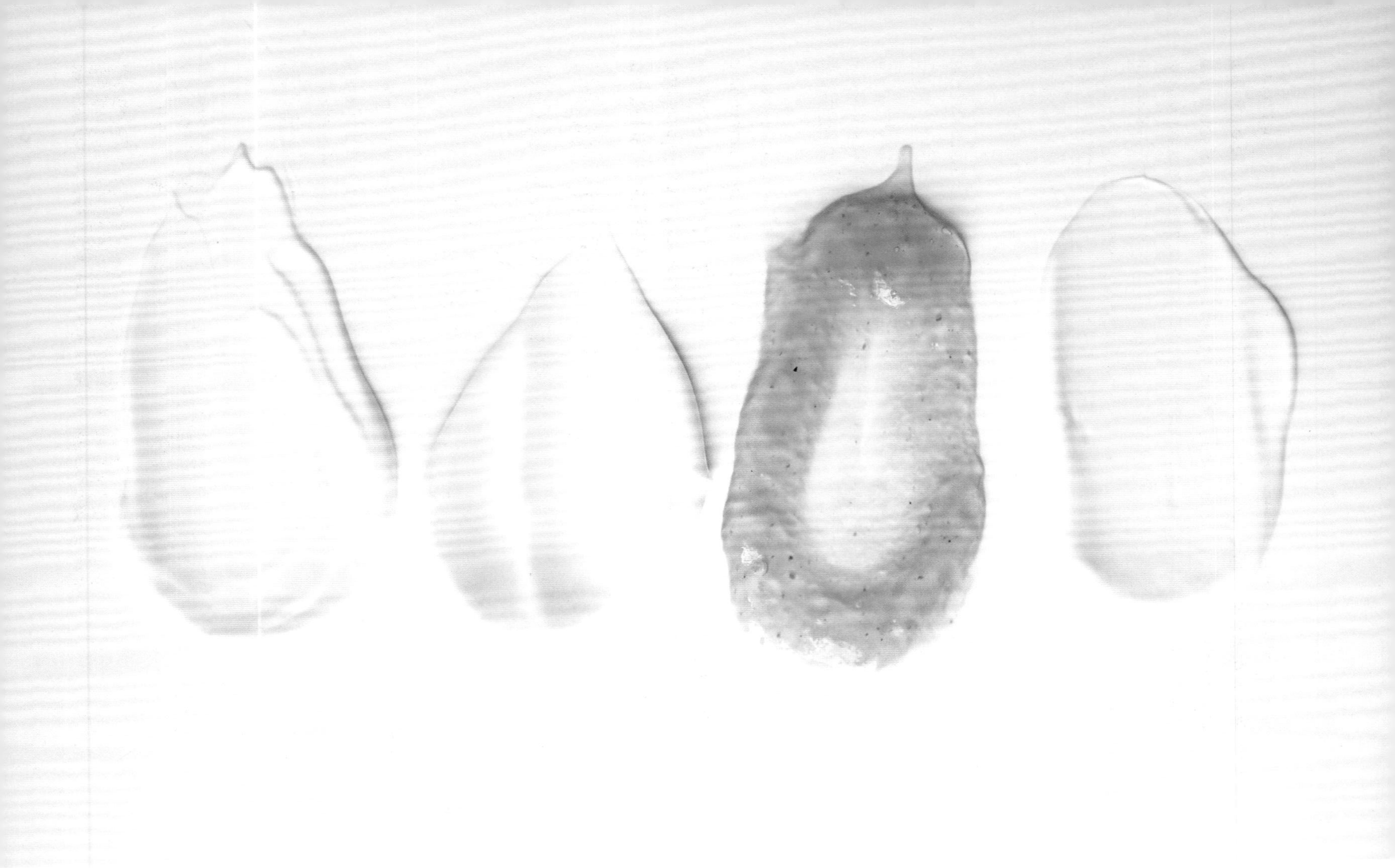

DECODING INGREDIENT LISTS AND CLAIMS

Now that you know all about skincare marketing tactics, let's get down to the formulas and what's in them, so you know what you're spending your money on. A lot of brands don't make it easy, but the ingredients list on any product is in many ways the most important part. Behind all the packaging and marketing, this little list is the science bit – it's essentially what you've paid for. But unless you're a cosmetic scientist or a trained expert, it can be hard to know what you're looking at.

HOW TO READ AN INGREDIENTS LABEL

The first thing to bear in mind is that **the ingredient (INCI) list is just a guide**. The true breakdown of the ingredients will only be known to the original formulator, the owner of the formula and the manufacturing lab that makes the products.However, if you learn a few key pointers, reading the list of ingredients on product packaging can still save you a lot of time and effort (and, potentially, money).

Ingredients are legally required to be listed in order, starting with the highest concentrate, until you hit the ingredients that make up less than 1 per cent of the formula. For example, in a moisturising lotion, you'll typically find water ('aqua') first, followed by things like glycerin, hyaluronic acid and, in richer creams, things such as shea butter, squalane and fatty acids. That is easy enough to understand.

The harder part is making sense of what comes in at under 1 per cent, because these ingredients can be listed in any order, and there is no legal obligation to list them in order of descending percentages. This is where brands get creative.

If a brand claims that a product has '25 actives!', I can promise you they will mostly be found under the 1 per cent threshold. This is such common practice that it has its own term – 'Angel Dusting'. Angel dusting is when brands add a miniscule amount of an active ingredient to their formulas in order to make grand marketing claims. From a legal standpoint, the ingredient may have proven clinical results, and it may be in the product, but there is no guarantee that there is enough of the ingredient in the formula to have said effect. That is the aim of the marketing and the assumption of the consumer. There are a couple of key things that you can look out for:

- **Phenoxyethanol or parabens.** Use the appearance of these in ingredient lists as a guide for percentages. Phenoxyethanol, along with parabens, is not allowed to be in formulas at an amount higher than 1 per cent. So, you know that anything listed *after* either of those makes up less than 1 per cent of the product. If a brand is harping on and on about their massively 'active' ingredients and they *all* come after phenoxyethanol or parabens, they may not be that 'active'. There will always be exceptions, such as retinols (frequently used at a strength of 0.3 or 0.5 per cent), but in general, you want peptides, vitamins and the majority of other 'actives' higher than 1 per cent. Mostly. It's not an exact science.

- **Alcohol.** If alcohol is the main ingredient in a product, or in the top three ingredients, I would expect the product to be perhaps an acid or an SPF where it can be necessary to facilitate the formula. You're looking for alcohol denat/denatured alcohol, isopropyl alcohol, SD alcohol or benzyl alcohol. In general, these alcohols are not great for the skin at high concentrations and I tend to avoid them.

FORMULA IS QUEEN – LESS IS SOMETIMES MORE

If you spend any time on social media, you will have noticed competition-level bragging from brands regarding the percentages of ingredients in their formulas. For example, 'contains 25% acid' and 'contains 20% vitamin C': nobody needs a 25% acid or a 20% vitamin C product on their skin on a regular basis. The ever-increasing availability of really high percentages of acids and high-concentration vitamin C products in particular has led to an increase in sensitised skins and the need for medical intervention and stripping back to solid basics.

The rise of single-ingredient formula brands and their marketing, while originally credited with democratising the beauty industry by supposedly talking straight and keeping things simple, in reality has given rise to customers buying multiple products, without proper guidance, and in a lot of cases ending up with 'Status Cosmeticus', aka Cosmetic Intolerance Syndrome.

There are good reasons that professionals would never recommend using a high-percentage acid, followed by a high-percentage vitamin C, followed by another 'active', such as niacinamide or hydroquinone. It's too much. Our skin has evolved over thousands of years into the perfect barrier. It will always win.

Stronger does not always mean better.
The formula is what matters.

WHAT DOES 'KEY INGREDIENTS' MEAN?

Key ingredients are the 'actives' added to a formula that have the potential to change the appearance of your skin. They are basically what you are paying for.

ANTI-INFLAMMATORIES

If your skin is red and aggravated, look for products that contain some of these ingredients:

- Aloe vera
- Azelaic acid
- Chamomile
- CoQ10 (Coenzyme Q10 or ubiquinol)
- Feverfew
- Green tea extract
- Licorice extract
- Niacinamide
- Oats
- Pycnogenol
- Zinc

ANTIOXIDANTS

Found in pretty much every product you'll buy (except for cleansers), everyone needs these ingredients because they help protect your skin from external pollutants and free radicals.

- Alpha-lipoic acid
- CoQ10
- Green tea extract
- Resveratrol

- Turmeric/curcumin
- Vitamin C
- Vitamin E

HYDRATION
If you are dry or dehydrated, look for moisturisers or facial mists that contain the following at the top of the INCI list:

- Glycerin
- Hyaluronic acid
- Squalane
- Urea

PIGMENTATION ISSUES
These are for brightening dull skin, and in strongest strengths are capable of fading pigmentation damage.

- Hydroquinone
- Kojic acid
- Niacinamide
- Vitamin C

PEPTIDES
If you're looking for an anti-ageing product (though I hate the term) look for the word peptide. Peptides are groups of active ingredients that do everything from aiding collagen production to helping smooth out lines. They are high-tech, not cheap, and you'll usually find them in abundance in serums, which is why serums are more costly.

ANTI-AGEING
Remember, old is the goal, but if you do want to tackle the signs of ageing, look for the following:

- Peptides (see above)
- Vitamin A (retinoids) – these are appropriate for all ages and skin types, but especially for those over 30.
- Vitamin C – this is vital in the skin to support collagen production and help strengthen capillary walls.

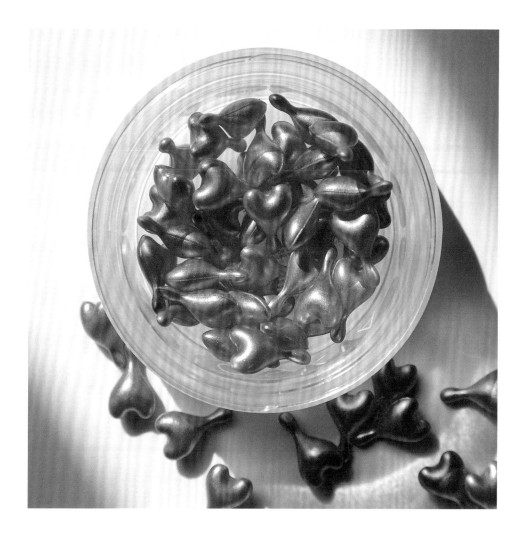

VITAMINS AND MINERALS

These are crucial in skincare so also get their own sub-category, as they can be found in most serums and moisturisers.

- Vitamin A – the aforementioned retinoids, and the gold standard of skincare.
- Vitamin B3 (aka niacinamide) – boosts ceramide production, thus supporting the skin barrier, and helps with post-inflammatory pigmentation.
- Vitamin C – the most commonly known of the vitamins, and the most thoroughly researched antioxidant on the market.
- Vitamin D – think 'defence'. Vitamin D is fortifying, strengthening and supportive of the skin's matrix.
- Vitamin E – used as an antioxidant and also to support and facilitate other ingredients, for example: vitamin A is shown to be more effective when used alongside a vitamin E product.

ACTIVE VERSUS 'INACTIVE' INGREDIENTS

What used to relate purely to ingredients that qualify as drugs is now used as a marketing tool industry-wide, and to say that the terms 'active' and 'inactive' are overused and abused by marketing departments is an understatement.

ACTIVE INGREDIENTS

When used in products that are considered drugs, i.e. SPF products in the USA (see page 155), active ingredients are loosely defined as 'any component of a drug product intended to provide therapeutic and pharmacological activity in direct effect to a diagnosis, cure, mitigation, treatment or prevention of disease, or to affect the structure or any function of the body of humans.'

Depending on what country you live in, retinoids, acids, and sunscreens like oxybenzone and avobenzone, are all considered 'active', active enough to change the structure of the skin. Take prescription-strength retinoids: in these, the vitamin A will be classed as the drug and therefore 'active', and the other ingredients are 'inactive' because they make up the rest of the formula and do not change the structure of skin. A lot of ingredients considered truly 'active' will have a maximum percentage that they are allowed to be used at in any formula.

WHAT ARE 'ACTIVES'?
'Actives' are ingredients (natural or chemical) that are biologically active and are typically the most potent ingredient in your skincare. They are put in formulas in order to remedy, change or target problems in the skin the product is marketed for.

INACTIVE INGREDIENTS

These are classed as any components of a drug other than the active ingredient. We are now seeing the words 'active' and 'inactive' used on product packaging and marketing material as a selling tool, not just in the case of drugs. A brand will say 'active' ingredients are peptides, vitamin C, seaweed, whale sperm... pick something. Anything. What they actually mean when they say this is, 'This is what we are charging you the big bucks for'.

Inactive ingredients are all too often completely glossed over, ignored or relegated to the very smallest font on the pack, and except in the rarest of circumstances, essentially mean 'the bulk of the product', i.e. water or carrier oils etc.

The potential problems arise when customers who are unaware of the above purchase something and assume that 'inactive' means 'has no effect on the skin'. Just because something doesn't change the structure of the skin (i.e. is 'active') does not mean that it does not affect the skin.

Alcohol, base oils, fragrance and silicones, for example, are all 'inactive' ingredients, yet the ones I am asked about the most by readers. You can bet that a high level of alcohol in a product will be 'active' on your skin in some way.

> If a cheese sandwich was skincare, the bacon would be labelled on the pack as the 'active' ingredient, but the bread would certainly be an active ingredient to someone with a gluten intolerance or a wheat allergy.

Ignore the marketing hype and read the ingredients label. That's where you see what is likely to be an 'inactive' ingredient that could actually be something 'active' for you to look out for.

Some brands have started using bold type for their 'active' ingredients in their INCI lists, in order to make them stand out. Clever, but not if you know what you are looking at.

PARABENS

I am asked on an almost daily basis for my views on parabens, the chemical preservatives used in cosmetic and pharmaceutical products, and am met with outrage by some people who are mortified that I am recommending something that is 'toxic' and can 'give you breast cancer' (erm, no).

In short, my response to the 'outraged' people is always polite and explanatory, but my response to websites spewing out this nonsense is 'bollocks'. They have a lot to answer for. For example, companies that rage about how untrustworthy the skincare industry is because it uses the term 'non-toxic' (because 'non-toxic' means 'absolutely nothing'), and then launch their own range of products described as 'non-toxic'.

I have no problem with short-chain parabens. They are not 'toxic'. I'm not a fan of the way that websites and brands in the 'clean' arena use that word for scare tactics or to make sales.

The word 'toxic' is always dose-dependent.

If a venomous snake bites you, you could die. If you take a little of that venom and use it to make an antivenom, it could save your life. It's no longer 'toxic'.

In a study of 20 women in 2002,[7] parabens were found to be present in breast cancer tumours. They were also present in breast tissue that had no tumours or cancer present.

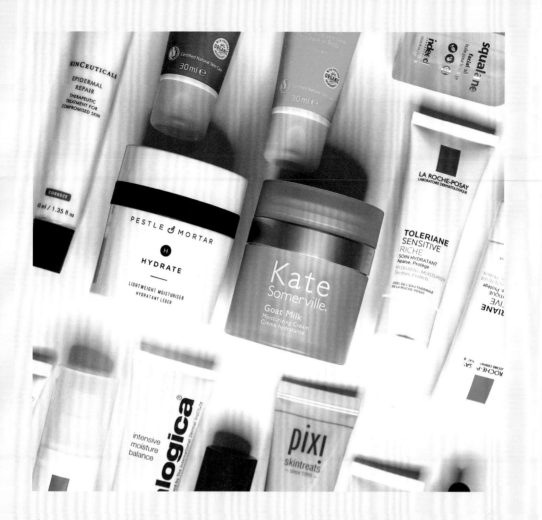

They are mostly present in your wee. That's because you break them down and pee them out.

I'm not a doctor and I'm not a cosmetic scientist but, tellingly, I have yet to work with one who has a problem with parabens in topical formulas.

While it's true that the USA does not do a good enough job of regulating the ingredients of skincare products, the FDA have done research on parabens and found them to be 'completely safe for use in cosmetics'. Similarly, the EU and Canada's governing bodies[8] came to the same conclusion.

If ever there was a case of the tail wagging the dog, this is it. The skincare industry has allowed scaremongering and marketing tactics from the 'clean' movement to lead, when they should have been kicked into touch by science.

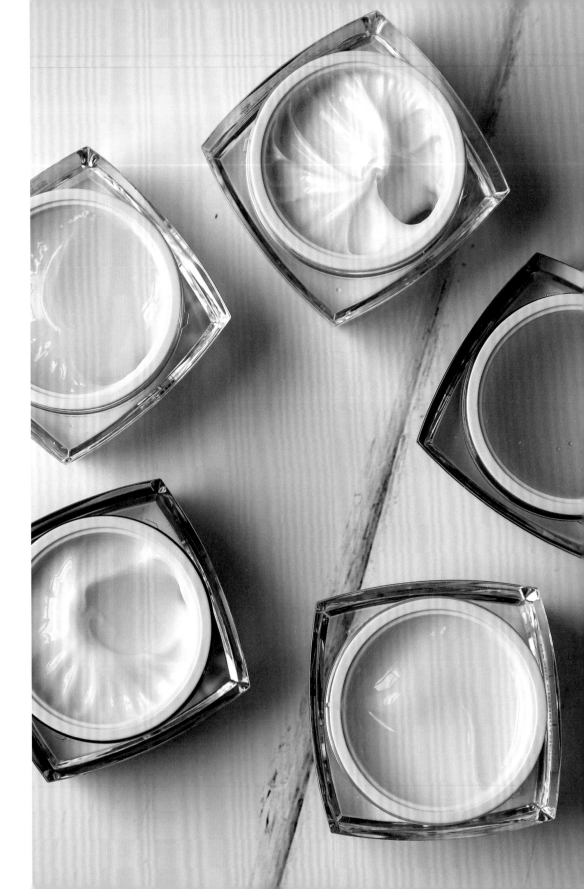

TRIALS AND STUDIES: WHAT DO THEY MEAN?

I am often met with claims of 'clinical trials' and 'independent studies' when reviewing skincare. It's to be expected. Brands want to give the consumer 'evidence' that their product does what it says on the box. The problem arises when they make those claims based on inadequate or irrelevant testing, and put the claims in language that isn't easy for the customer to understand.

So, here's a breakdown of what it all means, in its simplest form:

CONSUMER TRIALS/CONSUMER STUDY

You always see these in the small print on ads. They say something like: 'In a study of 80 women, 67% found that [X] product increased hydration in the skin.'

The major problem with these 'trials' is that you frequently have no idea of the demographic and skin type of those 80 women. If you put a really hydrating moisturiser on a 70-year-old woman who has only ever used soap and water on her face, she may think it's amazing. If you put that same moisturiser on me, I may think it's doing absolutely nothing.

Consumer trials, in a lot of cases, are really just marketing dressed up as facts. It may be a *fact* that '35 out of 50 women found that the product enhanced the firmness of their skin', but what was their skin like before? What is your base level in the group of women? How old are they? Were they wrinkled to begin with? Did they have acne? Did they have sensitive skin? We will never know. These trials are based on the participants feeding back their thoughts on paper, not studied in detail under a microscope in a clinic. That's a consumer trial.

CLINICAL TRIALS

These are, obviously, done in a clinical environment, on people, not petri dishes.

Clinical trials include monitoring the participants before, during and after use of the product and gauging results by scheduling tests, using equipment such as profilometry lasers, and strictly monitoring applications and dosages. During a clinical trial, participants following a protocol are seen regularly by research staff to monitor their results and to determine the effectiveness of the products.

IN VITRO testing ('in vitro' is Latin for 'in glass') is the most common clinical trial. The problem is that testing skincare in a petri dish does not replicate testing it on a live human being. Therefore, I tend to disregard any claims made in connection with in vitro testing. It's basically saying, 'This *might* happen if you use it on your actual skin! Or, you know, it might not.' It's the equivalent of Gordon Ramsay cooking an entire meal for you without tasting the food once during the cooking process. It *should* taste nice, but you don't know if it will until you actually eat it.

IN VIVO testing ('in vivo' is Latin for 'within the living') is the most reliable form of testing as the products are tested on people, not samples in petri dishes. This testing, however, is extremely expensive to perform and understandably not easily available to smaller brands who would struggle to find tens of thousands of dollars to test one product. Most studies conducted in vivo are limited to under 50 people – usually for cost reasons – and take place during a period of 4–12 weeks. For the simple fact that it is testing done on living, breathing human skin, it's still the most reliable form of skincare testing.

So, where does that leave you and I, the consumers who part with their hard-earned cash?

While I always take the results of a full clinical trial seriously, honestly, the only voice I listen to these days is word-of-mouth. If a friend has used something and really rates it, I want to check it out. If another colleague in the industry whose opinion I respect raves about something, I *always* want to check it out.

STEM-CELL PRODUCTS

stem cell
noun
   an undifferentiated cell that gives rise to specialised cells, such as blood cells

There are a lot of 'stem-cell' products around these days. Brands need to be very careful what claims they make when they suggest that a plant stem cell – a PLANT stem cell – can affect the cells in human skin. They can't.

> It's one thing to use peptides to stimulate and give a 'kick' to the skin and collagen; it's another to suggest that those carnations you bought from the petrol garage can reverse ageing and 'wake up' dead cells.

Medical research about stem cells always refers to stem cells that come from human tissue, but plant-derived stem cells are used in skincare products. It is illegal in the EU to use any human-derived tissue or fluid in cosmetics.

Plant stem cells cannot and do not influence stem cells in human skin.

If we could 'wake up' anything 'dead' or 'non-responsive' in the human body, don't you think scientists would use that knowledge to help people who are paralysed? Please.

'PROFESSIONAL'- AND 'CLINICAL'-STRENGTH PRODUCTS

The current trend of products that are sold in high-street skincare retailers and department stores being marketed as 'professional-strength' or 'clinical' is at best disingenuous, and at worst insulting to the intelligence of both the customer and the trained professional. This claim is mainly used when a product contains stronger active ingredients such as acids and retinoids.

Let's look at peels as an example. True 'professional'- or 'clinical'- grade peels are only sold to qualified, verified and licensed aestheticians and clinics. Those products are not safe in the hands of the untrained consumer. The true professional brands want to see your qualifications, your licence and proof of your liability insurance.

If I perform a modified Jessner peel on a client, the PH is **1.5**. A 10 per cent salicylic peel is **1.8**.

You would never perform that strength of peel three times a week, as is advised with a lot of these products found in traditional beauty hall settings. We find ourselves in a situation where we have brands that do not have any skincare-qualified people at the helm of the company, making 'professional-grade' products.

Using 'professional-strength' or 'clinical-strength' on packaging is designed to give customers the impression that they are getting the same product and result that they would receive in a 'professional setting'. They aren't.

The same goes for products called 'facial in a jar', or similar. You cannot replicate a clinic treatment in one application of a cream or serum, and any brands telling you that you can are devaluing our entire professional industry.

THE 500 DALTON RULE

'The what?' I can hear you saying. As a consumer, you have absolutely no need to know about the 500 Dalton Rule. I'm merely sharing this with you because it's outrageous that some brands and websites continue to claim that 60 per cent of what you apply to your skin is absorbed. Cosmetic scientists, pharmacists, aestheticians, dermatologists and doctors all use this as a guideline. I always have the 500 Dalton Rule in my head when reviewing products and recommending what you should put on your face. It's why those of us that work in the industry as qualified professionals are able to collectively roll our eyes at some of the more ridiculous claims that brands make about their products.

The 500 Dalton Rule is the scientific theory that the molecular weight of a compound must be under '500 Dalton' to allow for absorption into the skin.

Our skin is formed of many layers (see pages 58–59) and these layers have worked together perfectly for thousands of years to form the skin and act as a barrier, preventing substances from entering the body, but this barrier is obviously not completely impenetrable.

Arguments for the 500 Dalton Rule are varied but specific:

- Most common contact allergens are found to be under 500 Dalton. Larger molecules are not known as contact sensitisers because they cannot penetrate the skin, so therefore cannot act as allergens in the skin.

- The most commonly used ingredients applied as topical prescription drugs are all under 500 Dalton.

- *All* known topical drugs used in transdermal drug-delivery systems are under 500 Dalton; for example, a testosterone patch clocks in at around 288 Daltons. HRT patches work in the same way – they are designed to deliver their component through the skin and into the bloodstream.

- While there are some exceptions to this rule, most researchers would suggest that anything intended to be used for medicinal purposes should be smaller than 500 Daltons to ensure absorption.

Here are the Dalton measurements of some key skincare ingredients:

WATER – 18 Dalton

RETINOL – 286 Dalton

RETINYL PALMITATE – 524 Dalton (This explains why products containing a lot of this ingredient tend to give you a short-term glow, as opposed to really helping collagen and cell turnover etc. It doesn't penetrate the skin.)

MATRIXYL (PEPTIDE) – 578 Dalton

GLYCERIN – 92 Dalton

LACTIC ACID – 90 Dalton

COLLAGEN – 15,000–50,000 Dalton

HYALURONIC ACID – 1–1.5 million Dalton

SUPER-LOW-MOLECULAR WEIGHT HYALURONIC ACID – 10,000 Dalton

ULTRA-LOW-MOLECULAR WEIGHT HYALURONIC ACID – 6,000 Dalton

The 500 Dalton Rule comes into play in the world of skincare in a few ways, but for you, as a customer purchasing products, just bear the following in mind:

- The formula and delivery system is key to the skin's ability to absorb effective ingredients.

- There is a reason most skincare professionals suggest spending the majority of your skincare budget on the 'middle' of your routine (aka serums), and the 500 Dalton Rule gives you some idea as to why: serums tend to contain the largest concentration of ingredients that come in at under 500 Dalton. You do not need to spend a fortune on an expensive moisturiser (unless you want to). While it may 'feel' nice because it is rich in texture and probably occlusive, thereby preventing transepidermal water loss (TEWL), ultimately you're paying for the name: the performance levels of a moisturiser do not vary that much across price points.

- The 500 Dalton Rule is a sure-fire way of putting a clear, scientific stop to the constant fear-mongering from the 'green'/'non-toxic' community, such as '60 per cent of what you apply to the skin is immediately absorbed into the bloodstream!' and other such nonsense.

" SKIN IS A BARRIER, NOT A SPONGE "

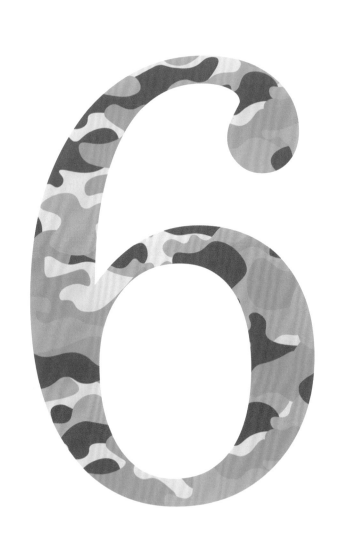

PUSH OFF A CLIFF

!?#

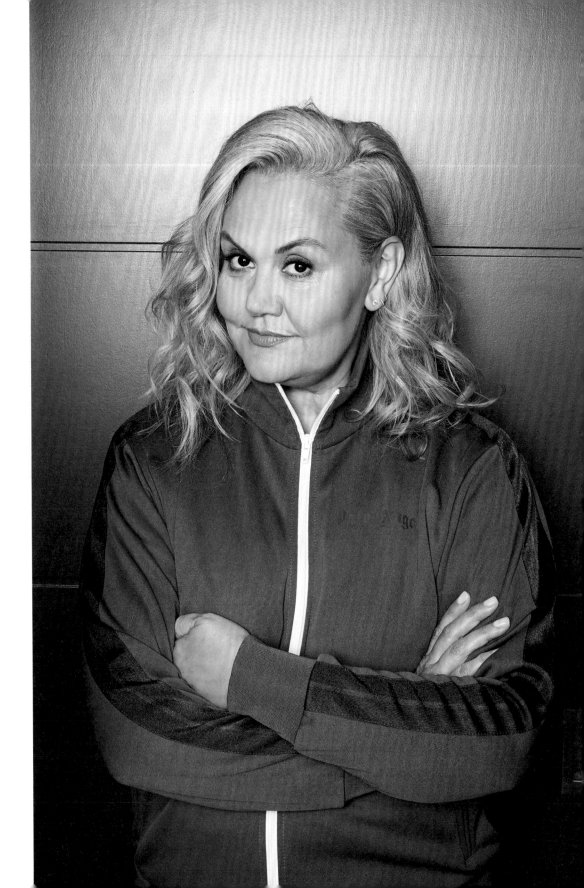

PUSH OFF A CLIFF

PUSH OFF A CLIFF

There are so, SO many products and trends that I would love to push off a cliff. Whether they're making unproven claims based on the latest buzzword bandwagon or just frightening you into trying to fix a problem you don't have, the skincare industry is rife with repeat offenders. I'm not singling out any particular brands here, but these are the products that have no reason for being on our shelves. Not. A. One.

- **Wipes.** They do not 'clean' your face. They are for Emergencies Only – real emergencies. If you have access to clean water, there *is* no emergency. They're also atrocious for the environment. Remember: Fannies, flights and festivals (see pages 168–172). And NEVER flush.

- **Sheet masks,** aka 'wipes with holes cut out for eyes'. Think of the environment if nothing else.

- **Foaming face washes that contain SLS/SLES.** I am not referring to the newer foaming cleansers that foam via a mechanical action on the pump, or are based around a gentler foaming agent. No, I'm referring specifically to anything that describes itself as giving you 'squeaky-clean' skin. No part of your body should squeak. These products are too drying. Full stop. You may want to also consider removing hair products and toothpaste containing SLS from your routine.

- **Micellar waters.** These are fine for removing eye makeup, or your entire face in an emergency with no access to water, but please don't use them without any other cleansers afterwards. Use them as a first cleanse only.

- **Pore strips.** I don't care who you see advertising them, no one who works in and on skin and cares deeply about your skin would ever – *ever* – recommend these. Horrible things.

- **Alcohol-laden, old-fashioned 'toners'.** It's time to move on.

- **Expensive clay masks.** Clay is one of the cheapest ingredients to put in a product. Don't pay big bucks for it.

- **SPF50 'drops'** that claim to give you complete SPF coverage, even when mixed with your moisturiser. Absolute nonsense. And dangerous. Don't believe the hype.

- **Harsh scrubs** containing 'husks' or 'shells'. There is no need to be so tough on your skin. It's not 1982. It's the skincare equivalent of using sandpaper to file a beautiful polished table. Actual horror.

- **Cellulite creams.** Cellulite is caused by fat cells pushing through your connective tissue. A cream will not fix it. Use a body brush and a decent body moisturiser. Your skin will feel smoother, but it won't get rid of cellulite. (See also pages 224–225.)

- **Gold in skincare.** Save your money. Wear it on your fingers.

- **Really expensive moisturisers that contain SPF.** SPF overrides any active ingredient in a formula. Don't waste your money. Buy a good, solid moisturiser and a separate SPF instead. Neither needs to be extortionately expensive. (See also pages 150–152.)

- **Glitter in skincare.** An oxymoron if ever there was one. Why? Exactly. Stop it. This also applies to anything that has a unicorn on the label. Gimmicks have no place in topical skincare (see page 142).

- **Coconut oil.** Although coconut oil has *some* antibacterial properties and can be used as a cleanser, any oil will take your makeup off. It's not the second coming. That's why it belongs here in this list.

- **Products sold using scare tactics.** Don't buy products out of fear. Certain elements of the skincare industry spend their entire marketing budget telling customers what is NOT in their products, and why they should be scared of certain ingredients, as opposed to what their products WILL do for them. Skincare is safe. There is no reason to buy out of fear.

- **Any topical skin product made using your own blood.** Taken from the idea of PRP (vampire) facials, founded by Charles Runels, the difference being that once your platelets are mixed in with base ingredients for a skincare product, they become completely inert, and are useless once outside the body. Also: illegal in the EU.[9] Fact.

- **Thinking that you have to use everything from the same range.**
It's a good selling technique to tell customers that everything 'simply must' come from the same range, but it's not true (see page 267).

- **Products that you have never heard of sold via social media ads.** Don't buy these. Remember those black peel-off masks?

- **Silly claims and extortionate pricing.** Brands that produce 'statement skincare', i.e. products that cost silly money for a 30ml of something with a huge claim attached to it, but no clinical trials to back them up. Nothing costs that much in skincare. Nothing. At least be honest and tell people they're paying for the packaging and your mark-up. If you can afford it and enjoy it, great. But if you can't, you're not missing out on anything that you can't get somewhere else for a fraction of the price. If you want leather upholstery and a better sound system in your car, you pay extra, but it doesn't make the car go faster.

- **Excessive layering of products.** I'm the first to hold my hand up and say I will happily layer two – *maybe* three – thin serums on occasion, but I am tagged regularly on Instagram by people/brands posting demonstrations of the application of five+ serums on a regular basis. Remember, you're talking about penetrating an area literally thinner than this –> ------ <– and only so much will go in. Save your money, use a couple and switch them up on occasion.

- **Skincare fridges.** Fridges do nothing to enhance the efficacy of products. They are completely unnecessary. All OTC products are tested for stability in extreme hot and cold environments before they are sent to market. However, if you like the feeling of something cool on your skin, go ahead – knock yourself out. But I'm assuming you already have a fridge for your food at home. Same thing.

- **Celeb- and derm-endorsed products.** Celebs endorsing products in magazines and on TV are being paid. So are dermatologists. Don't believe the hype. Do your research and go with your gut. Anyone saying, 'I only use this product and my skin is amazing!' is usually cashing a cheque somewhere along the way.

- **Mattifying products.** Unless you are a teenager and/or have oily skin, you do not need mattifying products. Healthy skin has a glow.

- **Be aware of dermatologists** recommending *only* La Roche-Posay, Avène, Cetaphil and Vichy (among others) repeatedly, and in isolation. Brands (French pharmacy brands in particular, in the UK) set aside huge marketing budgets every year to target and court dermatologists and pharmacies and win over all their 'affordable' recommendations. It's called '**detailing**' and is literally the skincare equivalent of lobbyists in politics. A full budget dedicated solely to wooing dermatologists, all so that when a magazine asks a derm what affordable product they would recommend they hear the magical, 'Oh, I always recommend XXX in my practice, it's excellent and does exactly the same as professional brands!' We all know it's not true but that's how the cookie crumbles. (That is not to say that some of these aren't excellent brands — they usually are, but when they appear endorsed by derms everywhere in magazines, someone has been paid.)

- **Botox parties.** Do not, ever, have your botox done at a 'botox party'. No reputable practitioner would provide this service in someone's living room where alcohol is being served.
    The first thing you should ask yourself when having anything done is, 'What would happen if this goes wrong? Can this person treat me for any reaction/bleeding/burning/bruising/misplacement/damage?' If the answer is not a definitive 'Yes,' then don't have the treatment. Simple. Legally, I could give you botox, but I would never do it. Leave it to the medical professionals.

- **Sunbathing.** More specifically, sun 'baking'. We need the sun. It's vital for our vitamin D. But we must respect it. Be sensible. Always use SPF and do not, ever, use sun beds.

- **Pore obsession.** Stop. They are never as big as you think they are.

- **Any pore-suction-at-home machine.** Save your money.

- **Smoking or vaping.** Stop. The end.

YOU HAVE TO USE EVERYTHING FROM THE SAME BRAND

I'm often asked these two questions:

'Do you use different products every DAY?' and 'Don't you have to use everything from one brand in order for them to really work?'

The answer is 'Yes'. And then 'No'.

Yes, I use different skincare every day, in the same way that I wear different clothes and eat different food, and I always have. Even when wildly restricted by budget, I would have at least two moisturisers and two or three cleansers on rotation. Your skin is different every day. Your products can be, too.

No, you do not have to use everything from the same brand. The only thing to be concerned about is clashing vitamin A products that you get on prescription, but in that case, your doctor would have advised you about what to use/not use when issuing the prescription. Over-the-counter products very rarely 'clash' because the percentages of active ingredients are low – they won't build up or interfere with each other.

What IS important is the order you use items and the formulas themselves. Your serum from XYZ won't know that your moisturiser is from ABC and stop working in protest. That's not how it works, no matter what sales hype you are given from the brands at a beauty counter.

The basic products I use, as a rule, tend to have ceramides, peptides and glycerin in them. They vary in strength and formulas, though may have similar ingredients. There are thousands of products out there. Embrace them (again, obviously within your budget), and the next time someone tells you that you simply have to use their moisturiser on top of their serum or they won't work, don't buy either of them.

WHY I DO NOT LIKE ELECTRONIC CLEANSING BRUSHES

Electronic cleansing brushes, also known as facial brushes, are a so-called 'beauty tool' that have rotating heads and exfoliate and 'deep clean' the skin. Where to begin on why **I'm not a fan.**

- **Because your skin is delicate.** It does not need a sandblaster to cleanse it. You have hands – use them. (If you don't have two hands, obviously do whatever you have to do and ignore this.)

- **Because they are capable of basically destroying your acid mantle.** Do you think your skin is 'purging'? It's not *purging*; it's inflamed. It's shouting at you, begging you to stop whatever it is you're doing to it. Stop it. If you were using a moisturiser that made your face break out into acne you'd be horrified, utterly horrified. And you would, in all likelihood, stop using it immediately and return it, especially if that cream was extortionate. But don't worry! In the case of 'purging', they have a brilliant idea! 'Buy another head'! 'You must just need something a bit more delicate'. Note how they've made it your fault. *Your* problem. And the solution? Spend more money. It's genius, if you think about it.

- **They are often aimed at people with acne.** The fact that these are ever aimed at people with acne is enough to make me feel slightly nauseous. 'Hey, you know what's great for acne? Using a power brush to really make sure the skin is as sore as possible! Brilliant! Let's do that.' No. Please do not.

- **Lack of training when the item is sold.** You can buy the most famous version of these brushes online. Just get it delivered to you, with no human contact from a trained professional advising you on how to use it. Which leads to...

- **People using them incorrectly.** I find, when talking to readers and clients, that these 'tools' are, without doubt, the ones that are most frequently abused.

- **The dirty head.** How many of you wash the brush head properly? Don't tell me 'It dries out and therefore the bacteria die'. Imagine using the same flannel for 2 weeks and never washing it. You can by all means let it 'dry out' between uses if that image makes you feel better, but imagine it. Filth.

- **The cleansers that the original version of these are sold with are 100 per cent horrific.** Horrific. I cannot stress enough how much these should be avoided. I promise you, the thought behind this was, 'How can we make more money?', 'Oh, I know! Let's make our own product! We'll say that it's the only thing people should use with them. OMG that's genius!' This was not a decision made for the benefit of your skin. A foaming, SLS-laden soap with a rotating (oscillating – whatever) power-blaster? In some cases, with grit?

It's like they sat together around a table and said, 'What could we possibly make that could irritate the skin more than say, oh, I don't know, wire wool and washing-up liquid?'

WHY ARE THEY SO POPULAR?

The popularity of these cleansing brushes is down to numerous factors:

- Because of the timer system, in some cases it will be the first time that some people have thoroughly cleansed their face. If you massaged a cleansing product into your skin with your hands for a full minute and removed it with a flannel after years of splashing off regular milks/gels, your skin would feel the same way.

- If you've never used flannels and acid toners, these brushes will without doubt exfoliate your skin. The first time you use it you will feel like your skin can 'breathe' properly. That's nothing you can't achieve with product and hands (and without sanding your face).

- Marketing. Your mate has one, it's all over the press, you WANT it. 'Oh, look, A PINK ONE!' *man voice* 'OH, LOOK! A black one!'

- And why is it all over the press? Because they make money. BIG, BIG, BIG money for the companies that sell them. Not just the brands; the retailers. If you go into a store and someone tries to sell you this, I promise you they are trying to make their target for the day. They may not have even asked you what skin type you have before they've said, 'Oh, you know what YOU need?!'

BUT: you don't have to listen to me. I know some of you swear by them. Good for you. As I always say, if it ain't broke, don't fix it. And do not stop using something you love on my account. If, however, you have a facial brush sitting in your cupboard that you shelved because it didn't agree with your skin, dig it out. Use it on your feet. Or your bum. Lovely.

I do think that, in years to come, we will see an increase in broken capillaries, stubborn 'bumps' that don't come to a head and rosacea, and I think this will be related to the use of these 'brushes'.

> If you suffer from eczema, acne or rosacea, for the love of ALL THAT IS SANITY, you have no business blasting your face to kingdom come with these things. No matter what any salesperson says.

You overuse facial tools. A lot of you. You can use them – you're just not meant to use them every time you brush your teeth.

Step away from the trendy facial tool and just wash your face properly.

And while I'm on things I don't like, let me give a special mention to jade rollers (or any type of mineral/crystal rollers). If they make you sit still and chill out while you massage your jawline for 10 minutes, crack on. They won't harm you. But, if you are buying one because the brand says that 'Once rubbed onto the skin, it increases circulation and gives a dewy glow,' or a 'lift', save your cash.

SKINCARE MYTH

!?#

WAITING LISTS

You know the things. Those long lists that retailers circulate, stating that 'literally thousands' of people are 'eagerly awaiting!' a product. Check out the press most days and you'll see plenty of articles about the latest one.

Here's the thing.

They do not exist. At least not in the way that they are portrayed.

Take it from someone who's spent her life in retail: there is no such thing as a list of thousands of people's names, all of whom are eagerly awaiting whatever product that marketing company is being paid to push that week.

> It's all hype, to make you want the product more and keep up with the Joneses.

In the case of something like the latest iPhone, with 10 million sold in the first weekend of sales, the majority on pre-order (i.e. already bought and paid for), the 'waiting list' is a legitimate claim. It's fact. If a skincare product is sold on pre-order and you pay for it, that's technically a waiting list. The rest is marketing. If a skincare product is really as 'wanted' as that, release it to market, let it genuinely sell out everywhere and spread via word of mouth.

Stop the nonsense.

DUPES

Everyone loves a bargain, myself included. Just make sure you are, indeed, getting a bargain and not being 'duped' into thinking that the cheaper version of a product is the same as the original formula. I can promise you that in the majority of cases, it isn't.

Read labels. That will help you find real bargains. Do you need to pay hundreds of pounds for a hyaluronic acid that contains one type of HA? Of course not (unless you want to, obviously). In that case a 'dupe' is indeed a good move.

However, if you're looking at more complicated products like acids and serums, dupes may not be all they seem. Most cheaper brands are purposely making knock-off versions that will include the key ingredient buzzwords from the original higher-priced formulas on the front of the packaging, but minimal amounts of the key ingredient in the product itself.

There are plenty of very affordable brands available on the market without resorting to the 'dupes' that are based on nothing but trying to rip off someone else's idea, piggyback on their success and in turn relieve you of your hard-earned cash for an inferior product.

'Dupes' belong in makeup and nail varnish. There is no 'dupe' for a high-quality, years-of-research-behind-it skincare product. Just because the packaging looks the same, it does not mean the juice is similar.

"

AN INFERIOR PRODUCT IS A WASTE OF YOUR MONEY, NO MATTER HOW MUCH OF A 'BARGAIN' IT APPEARS

"

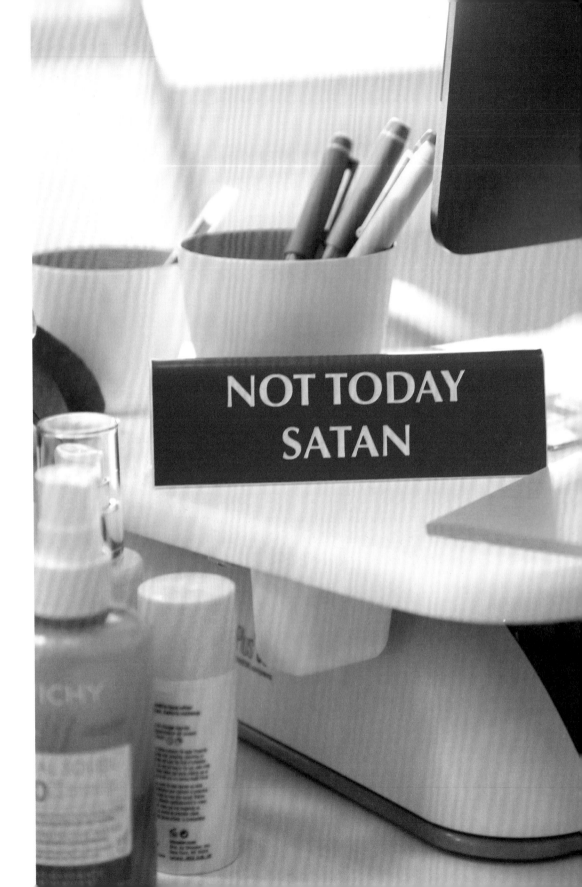

THE DIRT ON 'CLEAN'

The 'clean' skincare industry is worth a lot of money.

It's estimated to reach a value of $22 billion by 2024.[10] Over the past decade, skincare brands and retailers have adopted the words 'clean', 'green' and 'detox', and are throwing them around with abandon, fully suggesting that their skincare is somehow 'purer' and safer for your skin than a 'chemical' product, knowing full well that all products are made out of chemicals. If you know you're going to have an adverse reaction, avoiding certain ingredients is obviously completely valid. But the opposite of clean is dirty, and who wants their diet or skincare to be classed as such? Therein lies the selling power.

The entire 'clean' movement started in California and has spread, like an annoying, itchy rash, throughout an industry that has disappointingly forgotten how to lead by example and science and prefers to bow to marketing departments and the Environmental Working Group (EWG).

Some big brands and retailers have built their business on making you think that the skincare products sold to you can literally cause harm, based not on scientific fact, but the opinion of their founders, and more recently, shareholders.

We are now in a situation where the brands in the 'clean' arena use most of their advertising and packaging to tell you what is NOT in their formulas, while seemingly forgetting to advise their customers of what IS in them. As we've seen, you need to know what ingredients are in a product in order to make an informed decision about which will be right for your skin type.

They also bulk out the list of 'forbidden' ingredients by including things that would never be used in skincare in the first place, as if they're doing you a huge favour.

It is the skincare equivalent of saying 'There is no carrot in this yoghurt'.

This has led to the ludicrous outcome of the tail (customers) wagging the dog (the industry). It is both infuriating and upsetting to witness people with real skin concerns being told that they are somehow at fault for choosing to use products that contain the 'suspicious six' or the 'dirty dozen', or any other dramatically named yet arbitrary lists of ingredients.

'The good thing about science is that it's true, whether or not you believe in it.'

— NEIL DEGRASSE TYSON

Science and scientists are being ignored. Proven, legal safety assessments are being disregarded as if they are meaningless, and retailers are buying into it, heavily.

Since the first edition of *Skincare* was published, Sephora has now doubled down on their position on 'clean'. They described their new 'Clean at Sephora' seal as showing a product meets 'the strictest standards across the industry for clean beauty', whereas the reality here is that there are no standards.[11] No industry standard, and importantly, no legal standard.

This is ironic coming from a retailer that makes the majority of its skincare sales from the prestige, high-tech, doctor/professional section, none of whom would have ever considered calling themselves 'clean' before Sephora started putting the pressure on.

Allure magazine has the 'Allure Clean Standard'. Credo has the 'Dirty List'. (Yes, really.) Beautycounter have 'The Never List', which excludes nearly 1,500 ingredients from their products, yet they still use essential oils as fragrance — essential oils being one of the biggest-known allergens in skincare.

CAP Beauty store will only consider stocking products that are '100% synthetic free', which leads me to wonder how they are packaging them, but never mind. They also state: 'High vibrational beauty starts here. Let Mother Nature in and let in the light'. Ahem.

The Detox Market's top-line advertising declares: 'Green beauty brands to detoxify your life,' as if we are all bathing in arsenic, while Goop posts articles openly claiming a link between the 'toxic chemicals' found in personal care products to allergies, autism, ADHD and, horrifyingly, cancer, all without linking to scientific papers to back up their opinion, because at the time of writing there are none.

We as an industry have arrived at this situation because the myth continues to be repeated, unchallenged, that the FDA have no regulatory control over 'personal use' products. **This is categorically false and untrue** and repeating something as often as possible **does not make it a fact**.

The 'clean' industry, and it IS an industry, would have you believe that anything man-made is bad for you, and bad for the environment, and that for you and your family to remain safe, and free from 'toxins', you must stick to all-natural ingredients and use as few 'synthetic' ingredients as possible.

The irony is that they also link themselves to sustainability, something that is completely counterproductive to the 'green' and 'natural' movement. There is nothing green and sustainable about pillaging the earth relentlessly for 'natural' ingredients. Palm oil was once considered 'green'. Look where we are now. By all means use products with as few ingredients in them as possible, should you wish. Use products that contain ingredients mostly sourced from plants, should that be your preference. Avoid parabens (see pages 250–251) if you don't want to use them (but short-chain parabens are the safest and most-tested preservatives available). And eliminate all the 'toxins' you see fit from your life. It's 100 per cent your call.

> But know this: just because a product is labelled 'natural' or 'organic' does not mean it is better for you.

- The use of the words 'natural', 'clean' and 'green' is completely unregulated.

- Toxicity is dose-dependent. For example, apple pips contain amygdalin, a substance that releases cyanide into your bloodstream when ingested. Apples. Cyanide. Your body disposes of it. THAT'S ITS JOB.

- Every ingredient must go through a chemical process to make it into a product.

- Synthetic fragrances are known to be safer for the skin than 'natural' fragrances such as essential oils. They are also more thoroughly tested.

- OTC skincare (and makeup) sold via reputable brands and retailers **is not 'toxic'**. (I am not talking about 'preservative-free', made-in-the-kitchen-sink products sold independently or on open retailing sites, such as eBay.)

- There is no lead in your lipstick.*

- Deodorant will not give you cancer.

- Water is a chemical.

Charlatans will always try to relieve you of your cash. Do not part with it. You do not have to be 'scared' into buying skincare. Enough with the insanity. I love and use many a product owned by a brand that would place themselves in the 'natural skincare' arena, but I use them *despite* their messaging, not because of it.

*Actually, scientifically, there is the potential for minute trace elements of lead as a by-product to be in your lipstick as a by-product of pigment, but you would need to eat bullets and bullets of lipstick a day in order for lead to register in your system. Please don't worry. Safety assessments are in place, regulations are followed, and no one is trying to hurt you.

" EVERYTHING IS A CHEMICAL*"

*unless it's 'matter'. But you know, in skincare, we're dealing with chemicals,
no matter what the 'clean' industry would have you believe.

WHEN TO USE 'NATURAL' AND WHEN TO REACH FOR THE 'CHEMICALS'

One of my most-asked questions regarding ingredients is 'Is it natural?' and my answer is always: 'Yes, if that's what you *want*.' It depends how far you want to go, as all products sit somewhere on the spectrum of organic and chemical (and that's why I say a product is '-led'). See also 'Welcome to the Industry!' on pages 238–241.

Remember – everything is technically a chemical, including water. It's how a product is marketed that makes the distinction.

CHEMICAL-LED: products that contain non-'natural' ingredients – i.e. pretty much anything except a plant.

NATURAL-LED: products that would make the 'natural' consumer happy – they may contain some non-natural ingredients, but the main bulk is natural.

ORGANIC-LED: products that contain primarily organic ingredients, and usually list a percentage. They could happily be endorsed by the 'clean' brigade.

The best **eye-makeup removers**, such as those by Bioderma, Nars, Clarins and Charlotte Tilbury, invariably contain 'chemicals'. They remove surface junk, so

I don't have a problem with them. If you want to opt for natural, go down the almond oil route, but I find that a tad heavy for my eyes and the residue has the real potential to make you very puffy.

Cleansers/second cleansers are at some point going to be used for facial massage, so I steer towards good oils or milk ingredients for that. By their very nature, these contain both.

Acid toners/essences are, by definition, chemical-led. Lovely.

Eye products can be either natural or chemical-led, although I – as an older woman with visible lines etc. – would probably not go 'natural' here. Natural ones feel very nice on the skin, but if you want to fix fine lines, especially in the eye area, you need something made in the lab (which, of course, all 'natural' products are anyway).

Serums. I nearly always (and happily) use chemical-led serums. Here's why: if you are out of your 20s and have lived any kind of life (I *mean* 'any', I'm not being facetious) you will have signs of ageing on your skin. And I'm sorry, but at a certain point, if you want to reverse those signs of ageing, you need to embrace the chemical. For 'green' reasons, you may decide against that – that's 100 per cent your prerogative, obviously – but I have yet to meet a 'green, organic' product that can actually reverse sun damage, pigmentation and scarring as well as manmade molecules (think retinoids) do. As much as people harp on about rosehip oil for scarring, it has nothing, *nothing* on retinoids available on prescription. It may be marketed as 'a natural alternative to retinol', but in reality, that means that the proof has to be in the pudding, and they are just very, very different ingredients. This also applies to peptides (see Glossary), which are completely manmade in the lab, and are scientifically proven to have a very real effect on the skin.

Your serum is your powerhouse product – it has the biggest job to do. It's the most 'active' product that you will use in your routine. This is when you should embrace the chemical and be a bit more spendy.

There are days when I reach for something more organic in the serum department, usually when I want to get my glow on, just hydrate, or if I am using a particularly silicone-heavy moisturiser.

Moisturisers. This is probably the category where I mix up 'chemical' and 'natural' the most. I love organic/natural-led hydrating, soothing moisturisers. I like how the majority (not all) of them sit under makeup and I tend to use them on days where I am applying self-tan afterwards. The lack of silicone makes for better (fake) tanning.

If, however, I feel my face needs some oomph and a little kick, I would probably use something hi-tech that contains high-performing, active ingredients. For example: a Kate Somerville/Zelens serum under a Tata Harper moisturiser works a treat. Likewise, a Tata Harper serum under a Zelens/Kate Somerville moisturiser is also a good plan. I like to mix it up a little. The reason I invariably mix up the final two stages is silicone. A silicone serum, followed by a silicone moisturiser, followed by either SPF and/or a silicone primer makes for the higher possibility of 'rolling'. And I hate it when my products 'roll' (don't get absorbed and bunch up on the skin's surface); it makes me feel dirty, like I have to do my entire routine again. Weird, maybe, but that's just me.

ORGANIC: IS IT OR ISN'T IT?

I am regularly asked about 'organic' versus 'chemical', and the misuse of the word 'natural' (see page 280). Are the products you are using as 'organic' as they claim, and what does 'organic' mean, anyway?

At the time of writing, there are eight different certification bodies in the UK that give out organic accreditation, and many more worldwide. All of them have different requirements. What is organic for one may not be enough for another. It is as confusing as it is frustrating.

To the questions, 'Is it natural?' or 'Is it organic?', my answer is always: 'Compared to what?'

If organic is important to you, do your research thoroughly. You may be paying for something that came out of the ground or from nature, but if it did so via truly organic channels is open to question. Brands that are obsessively organic will tell you the how, why, when and where behind their products' creation. If there is no trail, I'd ask questions.

DETOX

The definition of 'detox':

detox *informal*

noun

1. a treatment designed to remove poisonous or harmful substances from your body, especially alcohol and drugs: *'he ended up in detox for three months'*

verb

2. to rid (the body) or undergo treatment to rid the body of poisonous substances, especially alcohol and drugs: *'he checked into a hospital to detox'*

Despite what the 'clean and green' industry would have you believe, we have our own built-in detox system. It's called your lungs, liver, kidneys and skin. Outside of the medically supervised detox treatment in a hospital or drug-dependency unit, any other use of the word 'detox' is disingenuous at its best, and absolute nonsense at its worst. And it has no business in either the food world or in skincare.

Detox products. Detox creams. Detox teas. Detox pads for your feet. Detox hair straighteners. **Enough.** If your body was 'full of toxins' you would be, at best, very ill and, at worst, dead. Brands: stop hijacking the word to sell more product. If you want to 'keep yourself as healthy as possible', then by all means:

- Keep hydrated – with water. Diet Coke doesn't count, people.
- Don't smoke.
- Exercise (or just go for a bloody walk/have a good regular stretching session).
- Get enough sunshine, or supplement with vitamin D.

That's all the detox you need.

GLOSSARY

Here are a few terms you'll come across as you enter into the world of skincare, along with some of my own favourites.

500 Dalton Rule	The argument that a compound over 500 Daltons cannot effectively penetrate the cutaneous barrier.
acid mantle	Your sebum mixed with your sweat forms your acid mantle, which is a very fine, slightly acidic film on the surface of your skin that gives you extra protection from bacteria and viruses etc.
acne	Or 'acne vulgaris' is a skin condition that presents as inflamed skin with pustules, papules and nodules. It is not isolated to teens and not caused by dirt. Hormones, genetics and your environment are the key factors here.
AGEs	Advance glycation end products – proteins and lipids in the skin that have been altered by sugar molecules bonding to them.
AHA	Alpha hydroxy acid (e.g. lactic, glycolic acid) – chemicals used in peels to resurface the outer layer of the epidermis via exfoliation.
alpha arbutin	A safer alternative to hydroquinone for pigmentation.
alpha-lipoic acid	An enzyme that, applied topically, acts as an antioxidant and is thought to have skin-calming properties.
angel dusting	The highly dubious pratice of brands adding minuscule amounts of active/expensive ingredients to their products to make big claims on packaging.
antioxidant	You'll see this word used numerous times in marketing (and in this book). Antioxidants are molecules that help to prevent oxidation – a chemical reaction that produces free radicals.
astaxanthin	A powerful antioxidant that can also be taken internally via supplementation.
azelaic acid	A fantastic ingredient used as a leave-on exfoliant, with proven benefits for acne skins and treating discolouration and/or scarring. Suitable for all skins.
bakuchiol	A plant-derived product considered a suitable alternative for vitamin A during pregnancy and breastfeeding, as it is shown to have a similar effect on the skin.

basal cell carcinoma	The most common form of skin cancer.
benzoyl peroxide	An OTC acne topical treatment, more popular in the US than in Europe.
betaine	A gentle hydrator.
BHA	Beta hydroxy acid (e.g. salicylic acid).
BHT	Butylated hydroxytoluene – an antioxidant that helps maintain the properties and performance of a product as it is exposed to air.
bookends	Cleansers and moisturisers in your routine.
caffeine	An anti-inflammatory – commonly used in eye creams for puffiness.
ceramides	Fatty lipids that help to hold moisture into the skin.
'chemical' sunscreen	Any SPF containing anything other than zinc oxide or titanium dioxide. Works like a sponge, absorbing and breaking down the sun's rays. Wrongly targeted as dangerous by the 'clean' community. Actually works better than a mineral SPF for darker skin tones and pigmentation, including melasma.
CIBTAC	Confederation of International Beauty Therapy and Cosmetologists – a qualfication for beauty therapists.
CIDESCO	Comité International d'Esthétique et de Cosmétology – international beauty therapy and aesthetics examination body.
collagen	The scaffolding of the skin and most tissue in the body. A protein that literally gives skin its structure.
comedogenic	Blocks pores.
comedones	Small black or skin-coloured spots caused by sebum blockage. Closed comedones = whiteheads. Open comedones = blackheads.
CoQ10/CoenzymeQ10	Antioxidant.
cosmeceutical	A made-up, non-regulated word that insinuates that the product will alter the biologic function of your skin. Marketing.
Cosmelan	An intensive depigmentation chemical peel, that includes an in-clinic treament and follow-up creams.
cryotherapy	'Cold therapy' originally used in skincare to treat skin cancer, now becoming more popular in clinics as a stand-alone treatment.
D2C	Direct to consumer – avoiding traditional retailers. (See also DTC.)

dermaplaning	A close shave on the face to remove vellous (peach fuzzy) hair, particularly around the jawline and under the ears to allow for better product penetration and give a good glow.
dermatitis	A blanket term for 'inflammation of the skin'. Atopic dermatitis = eczema. Contact dermatitis = allergic reaction on the skin.
dermatosis papulosa nigra	Small, benign lesions on the skin, particularly prevalent in darker skin tones
dermis	The layer below the epidermis.
DTC	Direct to consumer. Sells online, on sites such as Glossier.
eccrine gland	The most common form of sweat gland, found on all surfaces of the skin.
eczema	Or 'atopic dermatitis' – a chronic skin condition that causes itchy, red, flaky skin. Can be genetic but is caused by a mixture of skin barrier dysfunction and your immune system.
elastin	The protein that gives skin its shape.
emulsion	A water-based moisturiser.
EndyMed	Brilliant, minimally invasive radio-frequency in-clinic treatment for tightening and contouring skin.
epidermis	The outer layer of the skin, which is mainly responsible for a healthy barrier function.
essence	A modern take on toner. Usually a first step in hydration.
essential oils	Natural plant oils typically obtained by distillation.
EWG	Environmental Working Group – non-charitable organisation. Google it for yourself (it's entertaining).
extrinsic ageing	Skin ageing caused by your lifestyle: diet, environmental factors, smoking and sun exposure.
faradic	Face and body treatment using electrical muscle stimulation.
fibroblast cells	Cells that produce collagen and elastin, among other molecules. Found in the dermis.
fibrosis	When you have an excess of connective tissue, seen most commonly as scarring.
filaggrin	A protein necessary for the healthy barrier function of the epidermis, mutations of which are linked to a lot of cases of eczema and ichthyosis.

flannel	Small face cloth used to remove balm or cleansing oil (first cleanse) and provides mild exfoliation. Called a washcloth in the US.
fractional laser treatment	A laser treatment that includes microneedling.
free radicals	Unstable (altered) atoms that cause damage to DNA, cells and proteins in the skin.
galvanic	Electrical treatment to improve skin tone and elasticity.
glutamine	An amino acid that is a building block of protein, among many other uses.
glycation	Occurs when sugar molecules attach themselves to protein or fat in the skin. As collagen is a protein, this can cause the skin to become stiff and lose elasticity.
glycerin	A component found in the skin, glycerin as an ingredient is a must-have humectant that is suitable for all skins and ages.
glycolic acid	The mother of all acids, the smallest molecule, able to penetrate the deepest. Used to tackle ageing and acne, among everything else.
glycosaminoglycans	The foundation of the extracellular matrix, giving it structure. Key for healing wounds and inflammation.
GMC	General Medical Council (UK).
grip, not slip	How your hands should feel when you're massaging product into the skin.
HA/hyaluronic acid	Found naturally in the body and resides in both the epidermis and the deeper dermis, where it plays a key role in hydration and skin repair. It is able to bind moisture in up to 1,000 times its own weight when topically applied to the skin and also helps the skin heal after injury.
humectant	Used to attract and hold moisture to the skin.
hydroquinone	Used for skin lightening, to treat melasma and scars. Percentages vary worldwide, but in the UK it's capped at 4 per cent dosage.
hypertrophic scarring	A raised mass of collagen occuring after damage to the skin i.e. piercings, burns or cuts.
hypo-allergenic	Relatively unlikely to cause an allergic reaction.
ichthyosis	An inherited skin condition that occurs when the skin doesn't shed dead skin cells.

INCI	International Nomenclature of Cosmetic Ingredients (the list of what's in a product).
intrinsic ageing	The natural course of skin ageing, from the age of approximately 20 onwards (I know), but essentially the depletion of collagen in the dermis.
in vitro	'In glass' – testing done by scientists, in a petri dish.
in vivo	'Within the living' – testing done on living people (organisms).
IPL	Intense Pulsed Light. Mainly used for hair removal, pigmentation and broken capillaries.
ITEC	Qualifications awarded by the International Therapy Examination Council.
J-Beauty	Japanese skincare and makeup.
Jessner peel	Medium-depth in-clinic peel, consisting of a 14g/14g/14g split of resourcinol, lactic acid and salicylic acid in a 95 per cent ethanol base.
Juvederm	Injectable hyaluronic acid dermal fillers.
kaolin	A naturally occurring clay mineral, typically used to reduce excess sebum and remove impurities, that is the most common ingredient in non-hydrating face masks
K-Beauty	Korean skincare and makeup.
keloid scarring	Bulky scar similar to hypertrophic scarring that develops after trauma to the skin. More prevelant in the young and people with darker skin tones.
keratin	The protein that makes up the outer layer of skin, hair and nails.
keratinocyte	Produces keratin – the primary cell of the epidermis.
kojic acid	Used primarily for tackling pigmentation issues, it has been slowly replacing hydroquinone in OTC formulas.
lactic acid	A great beginner acid, and brilliant for dry skins and treating keratosis pilaris.
Langerhans cells	Your immune cells within the epidermis.
Laser Genesis	Non-invasive heat-based laser with a number of uses (it is mainly used to stimulate collagen).
LLA	L-ascorbic acid (vitamin C).

MED	Minimal erythema dose – the shortest exposure to UV radiation that produces reddening of the skin.
medical grade	More common in the US, this term actually has no legal standing. The only real 'medical-grade' products are prescription-only.
melanin	The pigment that gives skin, hair and eyes their colour.
melanocytes	The cell that produces and distributes melanin.
melanoma	An area of cancerous cells often caused by excessive exposure to sunlight.
mica	A group of minerals used to add glimmer/sparkle to products.
micellar water	Made famous by MUAs backstage – a quick makeup remover.
microbiome	The microorganisms that live on us (and in us). The future of skincare.
microcurrent	Microcurrent electrical neuromuscular stimulator.
microneedling	More commonly known by the brand name 'Dermaroller', medical needling is a popular in-clinic treatment that stimulates collagen. Be warned: it only stimulates collagen if you bleed, which usually means in-clinic and using 3mm needles. The at-home kits will not do this.
MLM	Multi-level marketing brands such as Mary Kay, Avon (originally), Tropic, Arbonne and The Body Shop at Home.
MUA	Makeup Artists
Nd:YAG	Laser used predominantly for hair removal and proven safe for darker skin tones.
niacinamide	Vitamin B3 – useful for enhancing skin barrier function and reducing uneven skin tone, lines, wrinkles and dullness.
NMF	Natural moisturising factors including squalane, triglycerides, cholesterol, ceramides and wax esters.
NPD	New product development.
occlusive	Blocks your pores.
OTC	Over the counter (i.e. no prescription needed).
oxybenzone	Helps filter both UVB and UVA rays.
panthenol	A humectant.
parabens	Synthetic chemicals used as preservatives in a variety of products. Successfully ostracised by the 'clean' community, despite being proven safe for use.

PCOS	Polycystic ovary syndrome is a condition in women whereby oestrogen, progesterone and testosterone levels are out of balance. This leads to the growth of ovarian cysts – benign masses on the ovaries.
PD	Perioral dermatitis, or 'irritating red rash around the corners of your mouth and/or nose that won't go away'.
peptides	In their simplest form, peptides are short chains of amino acids that are able to penetrate the skin and tell it how to function.
pH	Potential hydrogen – used to measure acid/alkaline.
PHA	Polyhydroxy acid. A larger-moleculed acid that penetrates more slowly and is thus suitable for most skins, including sensitive.
phenoxyethanol	A preservative always used at under 1 per cent, making it a handy guide for reading ingredients lists..
'physical' sunscreen	A sunscreen made entirely out of zinc oxide or titanium dioxide (or both), is referred to as a physical SPF and favoured, incorrectly, by the 'clean' community.
PIH	Post-inflammatory hyperpigmentation, usually caused by damage to the skin.
polyglutamic acid	Helps draw moisture from the atmosphere into the skin.
Profhilo	A brilliant newer form of injectable hyaluronic acid that not only stimulates your own hyaluronic acid but also has a proven positive effect on skin elasticity and collagen.
PRP	Platelet-rich plasma – originally used to heal sports injuries on the body, now used in facials. Not proven to be effective and I'm personally not a fan.
psoriasis	Chronic skin condition that produces dry, itchy plaques of skin and normally presents on the elbows, scalp and knees.
pycnogenol	Potent antioxidant derived from the bark of French Maritime pine trees, also proven to be excellent when taken internally.
radio-frequency treatment	Uses heat to stimulate collagen, elastin and hyaluronic acid production with the aim of tightening or 'contouring' skin.
Restylane	An injectible hyaluronic-acid filler.
retinoids	Vitamin A derivatives – the gold standard in true anti-ageing skincare.
rosacea	Chronic red, irritated rash with pimples that typically affects the nose, forehead and cheeks.

rosehip oil	An oil rich in fatty acids – good for dry skin.
salicylic acid	BHA – an exfoliating acid.
seborrheic dermatitis	Itchy, red skin found in the sebacious glands, mainly on the face and in the scalp, i.e. dandruff.
sebum	The oily substance containing fat molecules that lubricates and helps waterproof the skin.
silicones	Safe, proven ingredients used to both give slip and carry key active ingredients into the skin. Given a bad rap by the 'clean' brigade, unnecessarily so.
skin barrier function	You will see the term 'skin barrier function' mentioned frequently in this book. The skin barrier resides primarily within the top layer of the epidermis, also known as the stratum corneum or 'horny layer'. A soft, plump skin is a sign of good barrier function. A compromised barrier function will present as dull skin that feels rough and/or dry. Skin barrier function is vital for maintaining the temperature of the skin and protection against environmental aggressors, and maintains proper hydration in the skin.
SLS/SLES	Sodium lauryl sulphate/sodium laureth sulphate – foaming agents used in products like shower gels, cleansers and toothpaste. On paper, they're inert and safe. Upon using them on myself and clients, I have found them to be drying and, in the case of SLS, particularly irritating.
squalane	One of my favourite oils, suitable for all skins. Light and nourishing without stickiness.
squamous cell carcinoma	A non-melanoma form of skin cancer.
squalene	Check the label carefully – can sometimes be a non-vegan squalane.
Status Cosmeticus	Cosmetic Intolerance Syndrome – when you've used too many products and your skin has just had enough.
stratum corneum	The 'horny' layer of the skin – the area most affected by OTC products.
subcision	A surgical procedure using a hypodermic needle quite aggressively under the skin to treat acne scarring.
succinic acid	An antimicrobial and anti-inflammatory acid.

TEWL	Transepidermal water loss.
titanium dioxide	A physical sun filter.
tranexamic acid	Used to brighten the skin and treat discolouration.
triglycerides	Contains a high amount of fatty acids and is an excellent emollient.
turmeric	Used as an antioxidant and an anti-inflammatory.
ubiquinol	A derivative of CoQ10 – an antioxidant that reduces free radicals.
urea	A humectant.
vitamin A	Aka retinoids/retinols.
vitamin B	Niacinamide.
vitamin C	One of the most tested and reliable antioxidants.
vitamin D	Actually a hormone, but called the fortifier of the vitamins. Strengthens the skin and in your system is crucial for healthy bones.
vitamin E	The original antioxidant. Makes all the others, especially vitamin C, work better.
vitamin K	Frequently applied after treatments to aid healing and minimise bruising.
vitiligo	A skin disease caused by your immune system destroying the melanocytes in your skin, thus causing large areas of depigmentation.
wax esters	Component of sebum.
zinc oxide	A physical sun filter.

THE BRANDS

Here is a new revised and updated list of some of the brands and products that I am most frequently asked about. The list is by no means exhaustive, and does not include many well-known brands unless I am consistently asked about them (or one of their products). I have distinguished between brands that emphasise the 'clean', plant-based source of their ingredients and those that are science-led and talk more about the product formulas and results, though it's worth remembering that *everything* is a chemical, and everything comes out of a lab. Everything.

WHO	WHAT
AHC	Brilliant Korean brand, makers of the iconic Essential Real Eye Cream for Face.
Allies of Skin	Founded by Nicolas Travis, created based on his own experiences with acne.
Alpha-H	Great Australian brand, makers of Liquid Gold. Science- and formula-led.
Amanda Lacey	Founded by UK Facialist Amanda Lacey, each product is scented with natural essential oils and contains and plant extracts.
ANR	Advanced Night Repair, an iconic science- and formula-led product from Estée Lauder. Suitable for all skins, especially popular with 35+.
Anthelios	A popular pharmacy SPF by La Roche-Posay. Multiple options available. Science- and formula-led.
Arbonne	They have an ingredients policy where the first thing listed is 'pure'. They use some plant-based ingredients, but not a lot.
Aurelia	British skincare brand championing probiotics.
Aveda	The original 'natural' brand, except they really are ethical.
Aveeno	Brilliant, affordable body, baby and face care line from the USA.
Avène	French pharmacy brand that specialises in sensitive skin.
Avon	The first brand to put glycolic into a formula. The first MLM brand: 'Avon Calling!'
Balance Me	Family-owned British skincare brand.

Beauty Pie aka BP	A science- and formula-led beauty club with multiple levels of monthly subscription fees.
belif	Korean beauty brand that is a hit Stateside for Sephora. I'm a particular fan of the moisturisers – they're brilliant. They claim they have the 'best' and 'purest' ingredients, which gives the impression they are a 'natural' brand, but this is nonsense. (That's not an insult, just a fact.)
Bioderma	French pharmacy brand that makes the most famous micellar water.
Bioeffect	Founded in Iceland in 2010, Bioeffect is based on an engineered plant-based replica of EGF (epidermal growth factor).
Biologique Recherche	A French professional brand that makes the iconic P50 and some of the smelliest, yet effective, skincare on the market. Popular with older skins.
Botanics	Skincare range only available in Boots. Affordable, single ingredient skincare.
Bybi	Affordable London-based brand.
Carbon Theory	Affordable brand mainly focused on acne and blemish-prone skin.
Caudalie	French spa brand that bases its products on the power of grape seeds as antioxidants. Introduce themselves as 'paraben-free and natural' on their website (rather annoyingly, as I think they are more scientific than the impression this gives).
CeraVe	Lauched in the USA in 2006, CeraVe is based entirely on ceramides and replenishing the skin barrier.
Cetaphil	The infamous cleanser that is still, bafflingly, a top seller in the USA. In my opinion, water, three parabens, two alcohols and SLS do not a 'suitable for dry skin' cleanser make. But this doesn't stop it being a bestseller.
Chantecaille	Luxury family-owned brand. Science- and formula-led, with the levels of 'natural' percentages listed on packaging.
Charlotte Tilbury	Makeup and skincare brand founded by makeup artist Charlotte Tilbury.
Clarins	Family-owned French spa-brand. Science- and formula-led, with plant-based ingredients at the fore on packaging.

Clé de Peau Beauté   Luxury skincare brand founded in Japan in 1982.

Clinique   Founded by Estée Lauder in 1968, Clinique are mostly known for the '3-Step', which is a shame because they have far, far better products in their portfolio.

COSRX   Affordable Korean skincare brand.

Curél   Japanese skincare brand focusing on sensitive and dry skin.

Darphin   Launched by Pierre Darphin in Paris in 1958, Darphin is one of the brands that first made me fall in love with skincare. Botanical-based, science- and formula-led oils, serums, lotions, milks and creams, all layerable and made bespoke to the individual. Lush.

Dr Dennis Gross   Also known as DDG, a dermatologist based in New York.

de Mamiel   Annee de Mamiel is an acupuncturist, aromatherapist and holistic facialist. Her treatments are otherworldly and have to be experienced to be believed. Her science- and botanical-led product line is an extension of this, and it shows. Obsessive about ingredient sourcing (not an insult!).

Decléor   French-based spa brand owned by L'Oréal. Predominantly plant-ingredient focused.

Dermalogica   Founded in 1986 and now owned by Unilever Prestige, Dermalogica is an aesthetician-based brand with an almost cult-like following (not an insult!).

Deviant Skincare   UK-based 'skindie' brand. Their Cleansing Concentrate is one of my favourites.

Dr.Jart+   Founded in 2004, this extremely popular Korean brand is affordable and science-led. I use the Ceramidin line regularly. The brand name stands for 'Dr meets art' – it's not founded by a real doctor. The parent company was aquired by Estée Lauder in 2019.

Dr Sam Bunting   Dr Sam's skincare line is based around a simple routine with multi-tasking formulas.

Dr Sebagh   Based in London, Jean-Louis Sebagh specialises in aesthetics and non-invasive treatments. His product line launched in 2006 to huge acclaim. Originally trained as an ENT specialist.

Drunk Elephant	Hugely popular US-based brand now owned by Shiseido. Purveyors of the 'suspicious six'. They don't like me because I once gave them construcive feedback on their retinol (not a fan), after positively reviewing 11 of their other products. They call themselves 'clean clinical', so safe to say they place themselves in the 'clean' arena.
ELC	Estée Lauder Companies (parent companies of brands).
Elemis	British skincare and spa brand.
e.l.f Cosmetics	Affordable cosmetics brand based in USA.
Elizabeth Arden	This major brand celebrated its 110th anniversary in 2020.
Embryolisse	Founded by a dermatologist in Paris 1950, focusing on moisturising and nourishing skin.
Emma Hardie	Facialist brand. Formula-led. No mention of 'clean' (thankfully).
Environ	South African clinical brand, founded by Dr Des Fernandes.
Estée Lauder	The world-renowned brand was founded in 1946.
Eucerin	Affordable skincare brand formulated by dermatologists.
Farmacy	US-based 'farm-to-face' brand that is extremely popular with the Sephora customer in the US. Green. Very green. Take up a lot of internet real estate telling you what is not in their products.
Fenty Skin	Skincare brand owned by Rihanna, suitable for all skin tones.
First Aid Beauty	Skincare brand targeting specific skin issues such as eczema, anti-ageing, dry skin and acne while being suitable for sensitive skin.
Florena	Skincare brand focused on fermented ingredients.
Foreo	Swedish-based silicone cleansing tool/applicator that vibrates. A lot. It's literally a vibrator for your face. I'm not a fan. Again, not that this matters – they sell by the shedload.
Fresh Cosmetics	'Natural'-inspired skincare brand.
Garnier	French affordable skincare and bodycare, available pretty much worldwide.
Gatineau	Luxury spa and skincare brand.
Glossier	Online retailer, offshoot of Into the Gloss. Hugely popular with millenials.

Glow Recipe	Fruit-powered skincare from Korea.
Glow Tonic	One of the original acid toners, now in its 20th year. It's the Pixi product that spawned a multitude of copycat products and the overuse of the word 'glow' on skincare products by brands trying to piggyback on its success.
Good Genes	A hero product from Sunday Riley that uses glycolic acid in the UK and lactic acid in the USA.
Good Molecules	Affordable skincare line founded by Beautylish when Brandon Truaxe pulled The Ordinary from their site. Clever.
Goop	One of the worst offenders for using the term 'non-toxic' in the early days, and then fortuitously launching their own range, which of course is 'non-toxic'. Leaders of the 'clean' movement (that is not a compliment), but in reality their formulas contain high levels of alcohols, essential oils (and their allergen components) and would be classed as 'chemical-based' by anyone in the scientific community.
GOW	Garden of Wisdom. Ingredient-led, frequently single-ingredient led. Competition for The Ordinary.
Guerlain	French luxury brand that started with fragrance.
Hada Labo	Good, affordable Japanese range based on the benefits of hyaluronic acid.
Helena Rubinstein	The original beauty house. Helena Rubinstein founded her company in 1902, when Elizabeth Arden was 8, and 6 years before Estée Lauder was born. Coined the original three different skin types. Relaunched in the UK in late 2019.
Heliocare	Brilliant suncare brand suitable for all ages.
Jane Scrivner	Great independent UK skin and spa brand.
January Labs	Small, independent LA-based brand, focusing on simple yet efficacious formulas.
Joanna Vargas	Independent facialist brand. Joanna has clinics in NYC and LA, and specialises in hi-tech facials.
Jordan Samuel Skin	Independent Seattle-based brand – Jordan's also a true gent. Jordan and Josh epitomise the new wave of 'customer first' brands.

Josh Rosebrook	Founder of an independent LA-based brand and also an absolute gent. Science- and formula-led, with an emphasis on sourcing pristine, active herbs and plants as ingredients. For all skins.
Kate Somerville	The original celebrity facialist. Still based in LA and now owned by Unilever Prestige. One of my favourite people in the industry. Absolutely nothing gets past her – she's the Queen of no BS.
Kiehl's	An original true pharmacy brand, now owned by L'Oréal.
La Mer	Luxury skincare brand owned by Estée Lauder.
La Prairie	Swiss brand founded in 1931.
Lancer	LA-based dermatologist, founder of the eponymous brand and lover of a facial scrub.
Lancôme	Originally launched in 1935, this French beauty house is now owned by L'Oréal.
La Roche-Posay/ LRP	French-based spa brand owned by L'Oréal.
L'Occitane en Provence	French body, skin and wellbeing brand.
L'Oréal Paris Skincare	Affordable skincare brand with products split by skin type.
May Lindstrom	LA-based organic brand. May's organic skincare products are properly luxurious. May is also obsessive about ingredient sourcing.
Medik8	British-founded brand focusing on CSA: vitamin C and sunscreen in the AM, vitamin A in the PM.
Merumaya	Independent British-born brand based on products containing proven active ingredients at affordable prices.
Mesoestetic	Brilliant Spanish clinical skincare brand. Makers of Cosmelan.
Murad	Dr Howard Murad is one of the most respected dermatologists in the industry. His line is based around proven actives, and his philosophy is to 'eat your water' and reduce your stress as basic self-care for good skin.
Neal's Yard Remedies	Family-owned, UK-based skincare brand that helped get plastic beads banned from skincare.

NeoStrata	Originally founded in 1988. NeoStrata and Exuviance, its slightly more user-friendly diffusion line, were acquired by Johnson & Johnson in 2016.
Neutrogena	Mostly good, affordable skincare available almost worldwide.
NIOD	The more sophisticated big sister of The Ordinary.
Obagi	Originally founded by Dr Zein Obagi, a dermatologist in California. Dr Obagi now has nothing to do with the brand, but they still carry through the basic principles, which, in essence, are based on the belief that we over-moisturise the skin.
O'Keeffe's	Skincare for extremely dry or cracked skin.
Omorovicza	Luxury Hungarian-based skincare brand built around the healing properties of thermal waters.
OSKIA	British brand that describes itself as a 'clean, natural brand'. But don't let that put you off. Brilliant products. One of my favourite brands.
P50	One of the original acids on the market, made by Biologique Recherche, and truly iconic. Notoriously smells of vinegar. You get used to it. And it's worth it.
Pai Skincare	Made with sensitive skin at the forefront.
Palmer's	Bodycare with coconut oil and cocoa butter as the main ingredients.
Paula's Choice	Founded in 1994 by Paula Begoun, Paula's Choice champions a very strict set of guidelines for their products, all of which are based on key, proven ingredients. Paula hates essential oils like I hate wipes.
Perricone MD	Originally launched in 1997 by dermatologist Dr Nicholas Perricone, this is now one of the older derm-led brands. Dr Perricone is arguably more known for his anti-inflammatory diet advice and books.
Pestle & Mortar	Lovely Irish brand that make solid yet simple formulas that are affordable and work. Hard to go wrong here. Also they are lovely people (that is sometimes worth highlighting in this industry).
Pixi	London-born but Swedish-owned. Founders of Glow Tonic. Formula-led with some mention of naturals, but not obsessive.

Proactiv	Launched in 1995 and still one of the biggest-selling brands in the USA, mainly through infomercials. Famous for selling kits targeted to acne on a subscription basis. Not a fan – in my opinion their products are too harsh for the skin, especially the skins they are targeted to.
PTR/Peter Thomas Roth	Eponymous brand founded by PTR, who calls his line 'Clinical Skin Care', despite being neither a dermatologist nor an aesthetician. That annoys me. Can you tell?
REN	REN were one of the first 'clean' brands on the market (REN means 'clean' in Swedish). Now owned by Unilever. Science- and formula-led, and obsessed with 'naturals'.
Renée Rouleau	Texas-based facialist Renée founded her company in 1996 and is known for her '9 Skin Types', giving her consumer an in-depth online diagnosis tool that expands on the traditional 'skin types'.
Revolution Skincare	Famous for making 'dupes' of well-known and trending colour and skincare.
Rodan + Fields	Multi-level marketing company with the biggest-selling skincare line in the USA.
Sam Farmer	Unisex, non-sexualised formulations for adolescent skin and hair.
Sephora	Founded in France in 1970. Now the largest beauty retailer in North America and owned by LVMH. All-powerful. What they say goes, for most of the brands they carry.
Serozinc	A brilliant spray/mist from La Roche-Posay that contains zinc.
Shani Darden Skincare	Founded by LA aesthetician Shani Darden and home of Retinol ReformR.
Shiseido	Founded in 1872, Shiseido is now the largest skincare company in Japan and the fifth largest in the world. They own Drunk Elephant, NARS, Laura Mercier and more.
Simple	Affordable skincare geared towards sensitive skin.
Sisley	French beauty house. Formula is more important than naturals, but they do 'like' a plant: 'The best of plants for the best of cosmetics'.

SK-II	Originally launched in the 1980s and now owned by P&G, SK-II formulas are based around the extract Pitera, derived from yeast. Most famously known for their Treatment Essence and sheet masks.
Skin & Me	Monthly prescription skincare.
Skingredients	Young, Irish brand founded by 'The Skin Nerd' Jennifer Rock, based on proven key ingredients and excellent, solid formulas. The future of marketing, branding and messaging. Thank God.
Skyn Iceland	Skincare for stressed skin using ingredients from Iceland.
StriVectin	Brilliant science-led skincare offering targeted solutions for every skin type, tone and age.
Summer Fridays	One of the nicest brands to emerge in the last couple of years. Good, efficacious products with a beautiful aesthetic.
Sunday Riley	Eponymous brand from Sunday Riley, a Texas native with a focus on science.
Super Facialist	Affordable British skincare brand.
Superdrug	UK retail store with its own brand ranges such as Vitamin E and Tea Tree.
Supergoop!	Suncare brand founded by Holly Thaggard, after her friend was diagnosed with skin cancer. Absolutely nothing to do with Goop or Gwyneth Paltrow.
Tan-Luxe	The best tanning brand on the market. Covers every shade and every type of product for easy choice of application.
Tata Harper	Oh Tata. I love some of Tata's products – her cleansers in particular are amazing – but what I cannot handle is the fact that every product has '100% natural & non-toxic' on the front, as if other skincare lines will kill you. Good products, some of them great, but the messaging is off-putting. Properly 'clean', down to the packaging.
Tatcha	Founded in 2009 in the USA and now owned by Unilever Prestige. Tatcha is based on Japanese culture and skincare. Claims to offer 'pure' products. In order to get to the ingredients list on the website, you have to first read what 'isn't' in the products: a trend I hope will soon die.

The Blue Cocoon	May Lindstrom's hero product, and one of the most searched products on the blog.
The Body Shop	Originally founded by Dame Anita Roddick and now owned by Natura. The Body Shop was one of the first brands to embrace 'giving back', and it remains at the forefront of issues like sustainability, fair trade, being against animal testing and being a cause for good. Formula-led, although their USP is to base a lot of formulas around key plant-based ingredients.
The Inkey List	Launched in 2018 as direct competition to The Ordinary.
The Ordinary	Part of the Deciem group, The Ordinary launched to huge fanfare by offering single-ingredient formulas at cheap prices.
Trader Joe's (skincare)	For the most part, excellent, affordable, simple-yet-efficacious products. Always overlooked by the US beauty press. Their USP is to base a lot of formulas around key plant-based ingredients.
Tropic	Multi-level marketing range originally founded in the UK by Susie Ma, who sold a 50 per cent share to Alan Sugar after she appeared on The Apprentice (UK). The brand mainly talks about what's not in its products, and would absolutely describe themselves as 'green'/'clean'/'natural' (or all of the above). Its reps have a bad marketing habit of talking about their brand positively compared to others, which I am not a fan of, but they listen to feedback, which is more than can be said for a lot of other brands out there.
TTDO	Take The Day Off Cleansing Balm by Clinique – an iconic product, known by its acronym in the industry.
UpCircle	'Skindie' skincare that uses leftover ingredients such as coffee grounds.
Versed Skincare	Vegan and cruelty free, US-based, affordable skincare brand.
Vichy	Founded in Vichy, France in 1931 and now owned by L'Oréal, the brand's science- and formula-led products are based around the benefits of the thermal spa waters in the town.
Vintner's Daughter	A cult facial oil/serum that contains 22 'nutrient-dense' botanicals. Not cheap, but generally loved once tried. Fully at the front of the 'clean' world.
Votary	British natural-led brand founded by Arabella Preston and Charlotte Semler, based on botanicals, predominantly oils.

Weleda	Launched in Switzerland in 1921 and most well-known for the extremely popular Skin Food moisturiser. Green, plant-based. Science- and formula-led.
Yes To	An affordable skincare brand focused on single fruit and vegetable ingredients including avocado, tomato and cucumber.
YourGoodSkin	An affordable skincare brand aiming to help restore and maintain skin's natural balance.
Zelens	British brand founded by Dr Marko Lens, a consultant reconstructive and plastic surgeon with a PhD from Oxford and Master of Science from Harvard, specialising in skin cancer and skin ageing. Extremely science- and high-performance formula-led, but uses proven plant ingredients in all his formulas. I trust everything he makes. Dr Lens performed my eye surgery.
Zo Skin Health	Newish company founded by Dr Zein Obagi in 2007 (they obviously cannot use his name on packaging). They still hate moisturiser, though (see Obagi).

SOURCES

1　British Association of Dermatologists: www.bad.org.uk/skin-cancer/sunscreen-fact-sheet#applying-sunscreen

2　Canadian Government Health Dept: www.canada.ca/en/health-canada/services/food-nutrition/healthy-eating/vitamins-minerals/vitamin-calcium-updated-dietary-reference-intakes-nutrition.html

3　Journal of Neuropsychiatry: www.jneuropsychiatry.org/peer-review/depression-and-vitamin-d-deficiency-causality-assessment-and-clinical-practice-implications-12051.html

4　NHS: www.nhs.uk/news/cancer/vitamin-d-may-reduce-risk-some-cancers/

5　Diabetes.co.uk: www.diabetes.co.uk/food/vitamin-d.html

6　NHS: www.nhs.uk/conditions/vitamins-and-minerals/vitamin-d/

7　'Concentrations of Parabens in Human Breast Tumours', published in the Journal of Applied Toxicology (Wiley & Sons, Ltd.) and cited on www.dr-baumann.ca: www.dr-baumann.ca/science/Concentrations%20of%20Parabens%20in%20Human%20Breast.pdf

8　European Commission's Scientific Committee on Consumer Safety (SCCS) and Canadian Government's Safety of Cosmetic Ingredients

9　According to EU legislation (Regulations Annexe II, article 416), skincare products containing human-derived ingredients are actually banned in the EU

10　'Natural and Organic Personal Care on Track to $22 Billion by 2024', Global Cosmetic Industry, July 2016, www.gcimagazine.com/marketstrends/segments/natural/Natural-and-Organic-Personal-Care-on--Track-to-22-Billion-by-2024-3864954/1.html

11　www.instagram.com/stories/highlights/18120234508217240

ABOUT THE AUTHOR

With over 200 million views to her blog, Caroline is a fully-trained advanced aesthetician with over 25 years of experience in retail, including 24 in skincare, consulting and advising for retailers and brands in the skincare industry.

Since starting the blog in 2010, Caroline's no-nonsense approach on what you do and don't need to put on your skin has led her to be named 'The Skincare Queen' by her millions of followers around the world. Her loyal fans refer to themselves as 'The Freaks' and such is the strength of Caroline's knowledge, when she recommends a skincare product, it creates a retail stampede.

Caroline is obsessed with skincare – it's her business as well as her hobby. It's also in her blood as both her mother and grandmother started their careers working behind beauty counters. Never sugar-coating her opinion, her expert advice talks about the industry she loves and shines an honest light on products that really work.

Skincare went straight to Number 1 in the UK charts on its release, making it the UK's best-selling skincare book of all time. One of Amazon's best-selling books of 2020, *Skincare* went on to win the Lifestyle Book of the Year at the British Book Awards in 2021.

In August 2020, Caroline launched the Beauty Backed fundraising initiative to support those in the industry who were directly impacted by the pandemic and subsequent lockdowns. It raised over £600,000 in three months and an accompanying letter to the British Prime Minister gained just shy of 30,000 signatures.

With a lifetime of industry knowledge, Caroline Hirons started a movement and Skin Rocks puts a name to it. Launched alongside her blog, Skin Rocks is an edit and a shortcut, an education and a guide, a community and a movement. It's a natural extension of Caroline's personal brand with posts, articles, guidelines, how-tos and events.

Caroline Hirons has been featured in the *New York Times*, *Vogue*, *Elle*, *Elle USA*, *Harper's Bazaar*, *Bazaar USA*, *Grazia*, *Stylist*, *RED* magazine, *New Beauty*, the *Guardian*, *The Times*, the *Daily Telegraph*, *Stella* magazine, *YOU* magazine, BBC Radio 2, BBC Radio 4, BBC 5Live and is the resident skincare expert on ITV's *This Morning*.

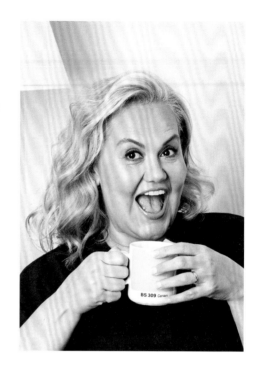

Born and raised in Liverpool and the US, Caroline has lived in London since 1987. She has been married to Jim for 27 years, they have four children and one grandchild.

www.carolinehirons.com

www.skinrocks.com

@carolinehirons

@beautybacked

@skinrocks

INDEX

309

INDEX

313

THANK YOU

The team at HarperCollins, specifically Lisa Milton, Kate Fox, Laura Nickoll and Louise Evans: thank you for your patience.

Megan Carver, Bev James and their brilliant teams, especially Aoife, and Becca, who herd kittens looking after me. Ten Forward Finance for keeping me on the straight and narrow.

Huge thanks also to my excellent doctor friends for their inside knowledge, advice and guidance: Dr Marko Lens, Dr Emma Wedgeworth, Dr Sam Bunting, Dr Justine Kluk and Dr Joanna Christou.

My 'keep me put together' team, especially Melanie Smith and Mercedez Mires. Huge thanks to my personal A-team: Everyone needs a LouLou Ellis, Christophe Robin, Molly Gyal Ting Hirons, Lucy Kids-free Kardashian Day Husband, Dominant Dom, Pummelling-the-back-end-Phil, Holly Victoria Barbie Brooke, Jill Marvel Mary Flannery, Katie George Michael Gardner, Josie 'the Vegan' Jakeman, Tasmania please-go-full-time Summers, Peter (poor Peter) Ade, Ashley 'Would you like the job right now' Horler, Lucinda 'not Megan's twin but totally is' Crowther and Alex Delightful Forbes.

What's for lunch?

Thank you to my family and friends in Liverpool, Warrington, West London and the States, and my industry friends all over.

Thank you to my family, all of whom supported me every step of the way: Mum and Steve, Dad and Theresa, Christopher, Michelle, Ethan, James, Heli, Lenni and Ted.

This book would not exist without my readers. Thank you, thank you, thank you for trusting me, challenging me, and supporting me. A special mention must go to the Skin Freaks group and @lizalaska who coined #carolinehironsmademedoit and started a movement that continues to astound me. THANK YOU.

And, most of all, to Jim, Ben, Lily, Dan, Ava, Max and the light of all our lives, Nova. All of this would be utterly pointless without you all. I love you.

HQ
An imprint of HarperCollinsPublishers Ltd
1 London Bridge Street
London SE1 9GF

First published in Great Britain by
HQ, an imprint of HarperCollinsPublishers Ltd 2021

ISBN 9780008517823

3

MIX
Paper from
responsible sources
FSC™ C007454
www.fsc.org

This book is produced from independently certified FSC™ paper
to ensure responsible forest management.

For more information visit: www.harpercollins.co.uk

Editorial director: Kate Fox
Project editor: Laura Nickoll
Page design: Louise Evans

Printed and bound in Italy by Rotolito.

While the author of this work has made every effort to ensure that the
information contained in this book is as accurate and up-to-date as possible at
the time of publication, medical and pharmaceutical knowledge is constantly
changing and the application of it to particular circumstances depends on
many factors. Therefore it is recommended that readers always consult a
qualified medical specialist for individual advice. This book should not be
used as an alternative to seeking specialist medical advice which should be
sought before any action is taken. The author and publishers cannot be held
responsible for any errors and omissions that maybe found in the text, or
any actions that may be taken by a reader as a result of any reliance on the
information contained in the text which is taken entirely at the reader's own risk.

All author photography © Nicky Johnston with
the exception of images on:

25, 28, 34, 48, 49, 51, 52, 61, 64, 78, 100, 104,
110, 119, 129, 130, 146, 159, 176, 187, 205, 211,
220, 223, 226, 238, 242, 247, 251, 252, 274 ©
Christopher Oakman

6, 162, 191, 202, 203 © Caroline Hirons

67 top left © Oscar C. Williams / Dreamstime,
67 top right and bottom left PeopleImages /
iStockphoto, 67 bottom right DUANGJAN J /
Shutterstock, 70 left Tunatura / Shutterstock, 70
right © Natalia Bachkova / Dreamstime, 71
Timonina / Shutterstock, 72 left YAY Media AS /
Alamy Stock Photo, 72 right sruilk / Shutterstock,
74 Mediscan / Alamy Stock Photo, 75 left
shurkin_son / Shutterstock, 75 right SCIENCE
PHOTO LIBRARY, 137 left BlurryMe /
Shutterstock, 89 Kanokpon Duangwaew
/ Shutterstock, 93 right Ocskay Bence /
Shutterstock, 94 Miroslav Lukic / Shutterstock,
96 vchal / Shutterstock

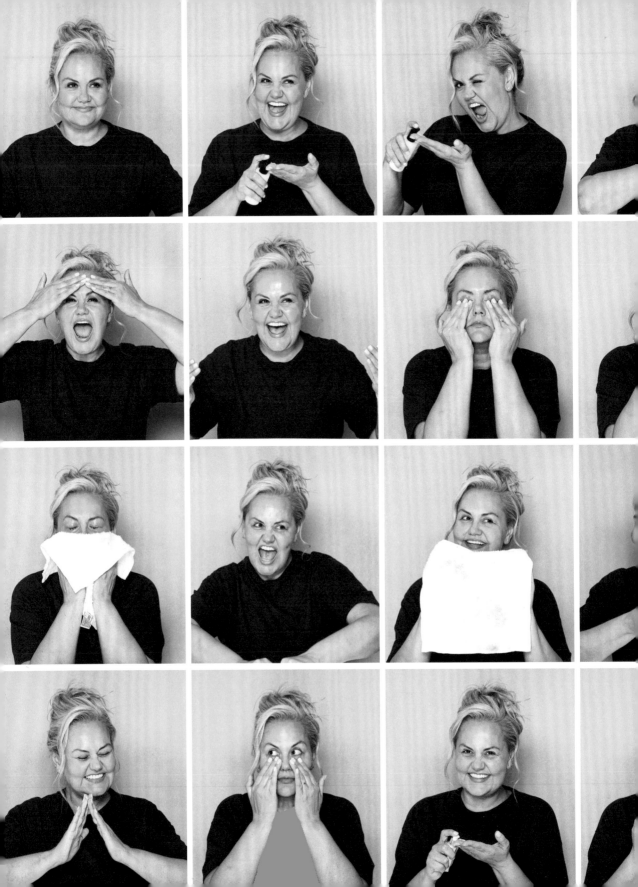